Rosa M PAL

DASH DIET MEAL PREP for Beginners 2024

The Guide to Cook Healthy Food with Delicious Low Sodium Recipes to Lower Your Blood Pressure and Meal Plan Preserve Heart Health

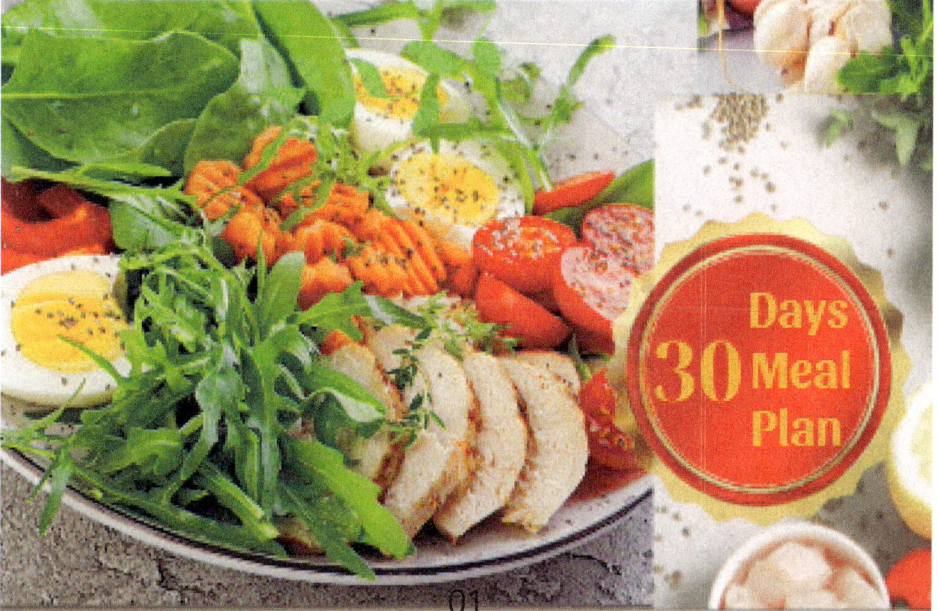

30 Days Meal Plan

DASH DIET

BREAKFAST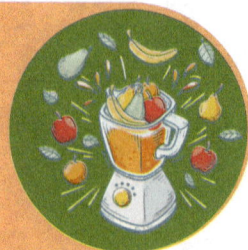

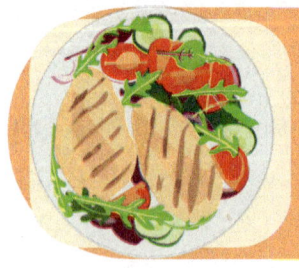 ## LUNCH

SNACK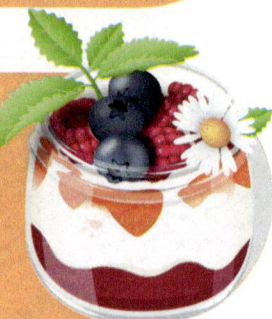

 ## DINNER

Cooking recipe

Spinach and Kale Smoothie

 Prep: 10 mins
 Cook: 10 mins
 Serves: 1

NUTRITION

- Calories: 325
- Fat: 14g
- Carbs: 46g
- Protein: 10g

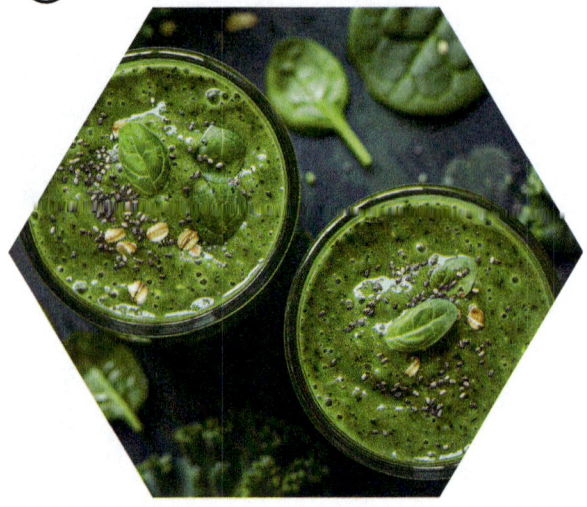

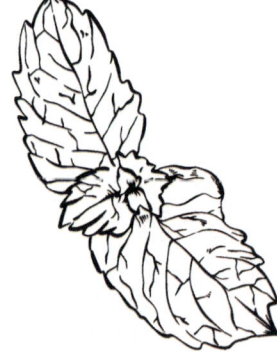

INGREDIENTS

- 2 cups fresh spinach
- 1 cup almond milk
- 1 leaf kale
- 1 tablespoon peanut butter
- 1 tablespoon chia seeds (Optional)
- 1 sliced frozen banana

DIRECTION

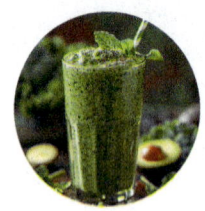 Combine spinach, almond milk, kale, peanut butter, and chia seeds in a blender; blend until smooth. Add banana and blend until smooth.

Blueberry Spinach Smoothie

 Prep: 5 mins

 Cook: 0 mins

 Serves: 1

NUTRITION

- Calories: 257
- Fat: 5g
- Carbs: 47g
- Protein: 10g

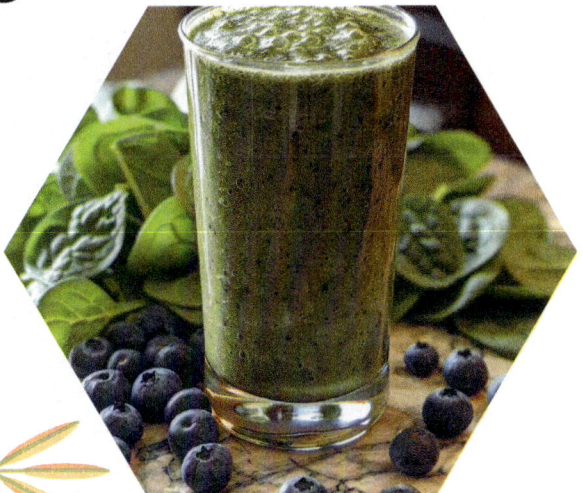

INGREDIENTS

- 1 1/2 cups frozen blueberries
- 3/4 cup plain whole milk greek yogurt
- 1 handful fresh spinach, rinsed
- 1 banana
- 1/4 cup whole raw almonds
- 1 tablespoon ground flax
- 1 pinch ground cinnamon (optional)
- 1 pinch ground nutmeg (optional)
- 1 pinch ground cloves (optional)
- 1 pinch cardamom (optional)
- 2 tablespoons milk, or as needed

DIRECTION

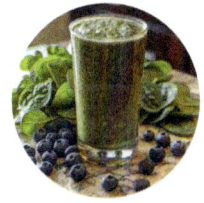

1. Blend soy milk and spinach together in a blender until smooth. Add banana and pulse until thoroughly blended.

Spinach and Banana Power Smoothie

 Prep: 10 mins
Cook: 10 mins

 Serves: 1

NUTRITION

- Calories: 257
- Fat: 5g
- Carbs: 47g
- Protein: 10g

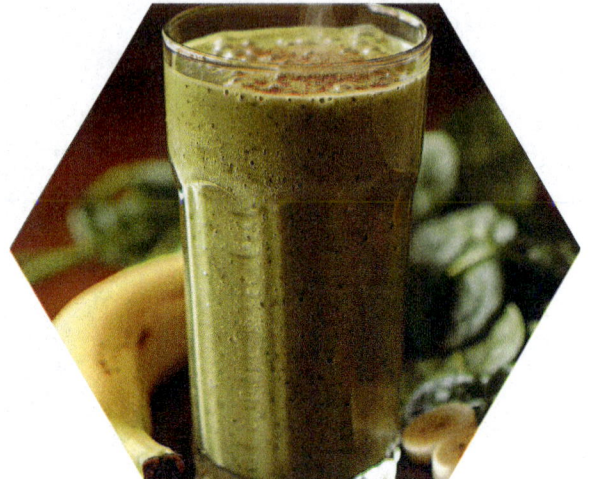

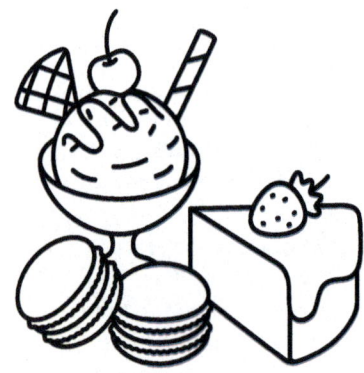

INGREDIENTS

- 1 cup plain soy milk
- ¾ cup packed fresh spinach leaves
- 1 large banana, sliced

DIRECTION

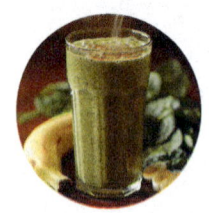

1. Blend soy milk and spinach together in a blender until smooth. Add banana and pulse until thoroughly blended.

06

Pineapple and Banana Smoothie

 Prep: 5 mins
Cook: 5 mins

 Serves: 1

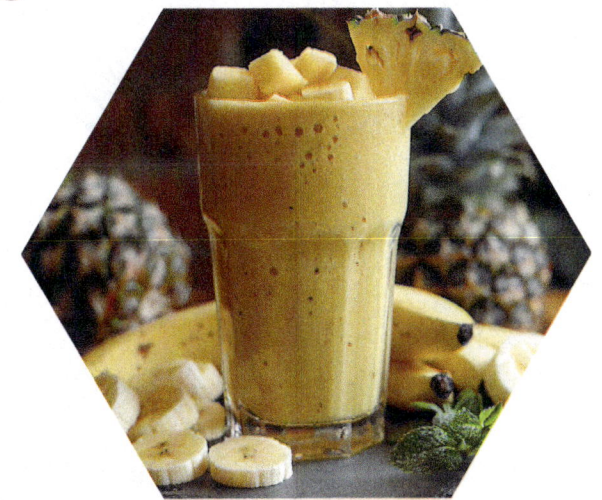

NUTRITION

- Calories: 313
- Fat: 1g
- Carbs: 79g
- Protein: 3g

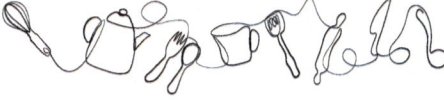

INGREDIENTS

- 4 ice cubes
- ¼ fresh pineapple - peeled, cored and cubed
- 1 large banana, cut into chunks
- 1 cup pineapple or apple juice

DIRECTION

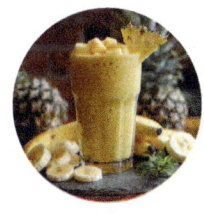

1. Gather all ingredients.
2. Place ice cubes, pineapple, banana, and pineapple juice into the container of a blender.
3. Purée on high until smooth.
4. Enjoy!

Strawberry-Avocado-Mint Smoothie

Prep: 10 mins
Cook: 10 mins
 Serves: 2

NUTRITION

- Calories: 353
- Fat: 14g
- Carbs: 47g
- Protein: 15g

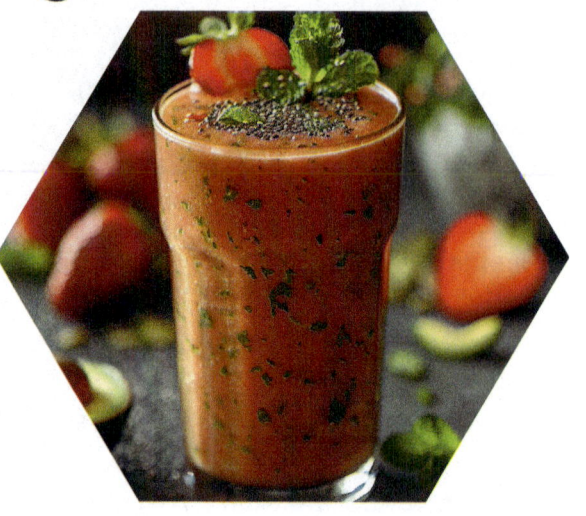

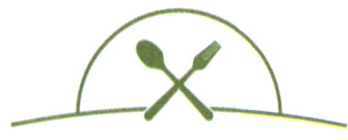

INGREDIENTS

- 16 fresh mint leaves, torn in half
- 2 cups frozen strawberries
- 2 (5.3 ounce) containers nonfat strawberry-flavored Greek yogurt (such as Dannon Light & Fit)
- 1 cup vanilla-flavored almond milk
- 1 small avocado, cut into chunks

DIRECTION

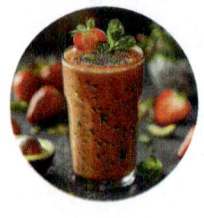

1. Place mint, strawberries, yogurt, almond milk, and avocado into an electric blender and blend until smooth.

Cucumber-Honeydew Smoothie

 Prep: 15 mins
Cook: 15 mins

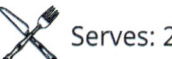 Serves: 2

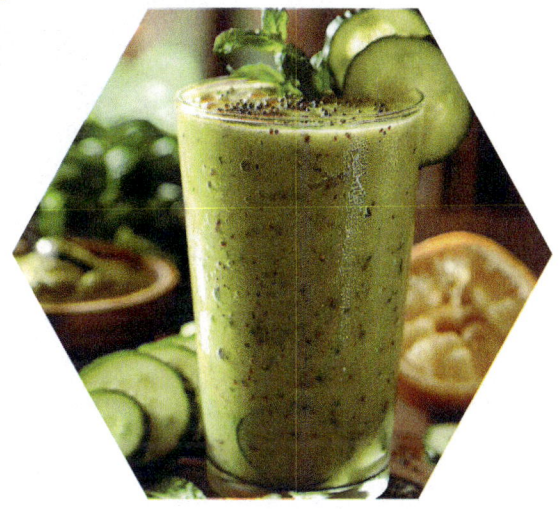

NUTRITION

- Calories: 237
- Fat: 1g
- Carbs: 58g
- Protein: 4g

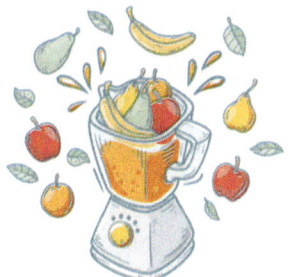

INGREDIENTS

- 1 cucumber, peeled, seeded and chopped
- 2 cups cubed honeydew melon
- 2 cups passion fruit juice
- 8 sprigs fresh mint, or amount to taste
- 2 cups crushed ice

DIRECTION

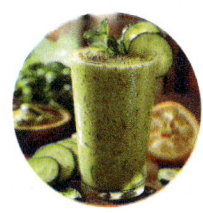

1. Combine cucumber, honeydew melon, passion fruit juice, and ice in a blender. Pull leaves from mint springs and add to blender. Blend mixture until smooth. Pour into tall glasses.

Mango Banana Smoothie

 Prep: 5 mins
Cook: 5 mins

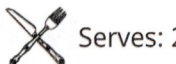

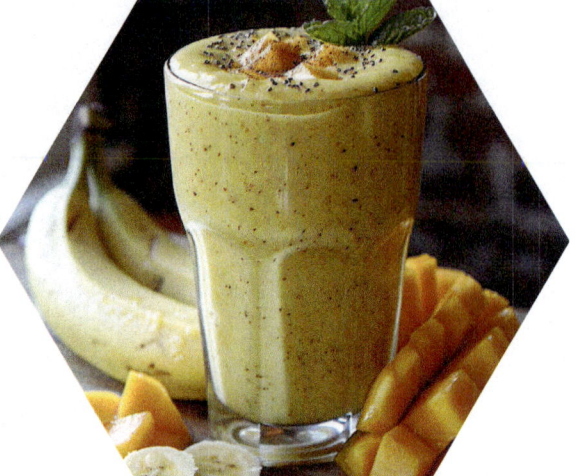

NUTRITION

- Calories: 135
- Fat: 1g
- Carbs: 30g
- Protein: 3g

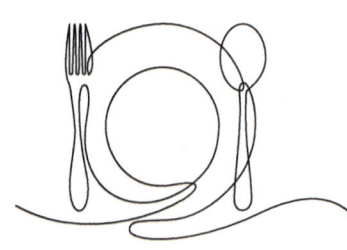

INGREDIENTS

- 1 large banana, cut in chunks
- ½ cup frozen mango pieces
- ½ cup orange-mango juice blend
- ⅓ cup plain yogurt

DIRECTION

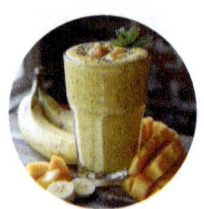

1. Blend banana, mango, juice, and yogurt in a blender until nearly smooth.

Bananerberry Smoothie

 Prep: 10 mins
Cook: 10 mins

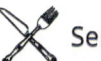 Serves: 2

NUTRITION

- Calories: 345
- Fat: 13g
- Carbs: 58g
- Protein: 7g

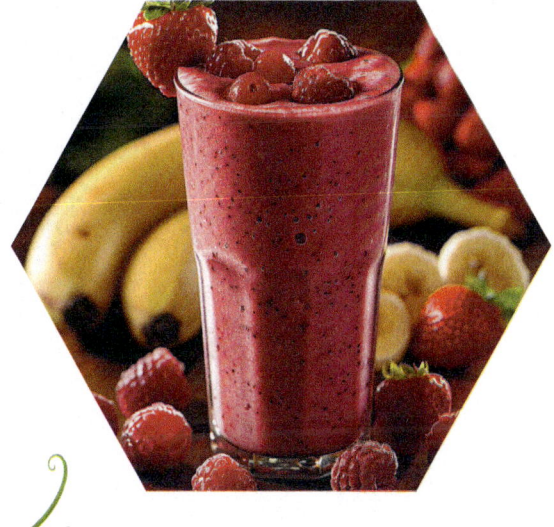

INGREDIENTS

- 1 cup fresh strawberries
- 1 banana, sliced
- 1 cup fresh peaches
- 1 cup apples
- 1 ½ cups vanilla ice cream
- 1 ½ cups ice cubes
- ½ cup milk

DIRECTION

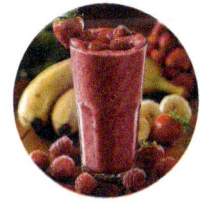

1. In a blender combine strawberries, banana, peaches, apples, and ice cream. Blend until smooth. Add ice, pour in milk and blend again until smooth. Serve immediately.

HEALTHY PORRIDGE BOWL

 Prep: 10 mins
Cook: 25 mins

 Serves: 4

NUTRITION

- kcal: 533
- fat: 19g
- saturates: 3g
- carbs: 66g
- sugars: 14g
- fibre: 13g
- protein: 17g
- salt: 0.1g

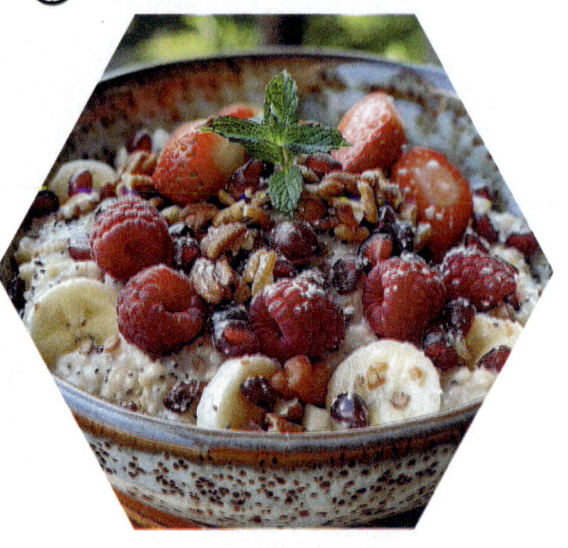

INGREDIENTS

- 100g frozen raspberries
- 1 orange, ½ sliced and ½ juiced
- 150g porridge oats
- 100ml milk
- ½ banana, sliced
- 2 tbsp smooth almond butter
- 1 tbsp goji berries

1 tbsp chia seeds

DIRECTION

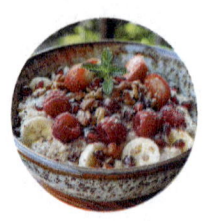

1. Step 1: Combine half of the raspberries and all of the orange juice in a pan. Simmer until the raspberries soften, about 5 minutes.
2. Step 2: Meanwhile, stir oats, milk, and 450ml water in a pan over low heat until creamy. Top with the raspberry compote, remaining raspberries, orange slices, banana, almond butter, goji berries, and chia seeds.

HEALTHY GRANOLA

 Prep: 5 mins
Cook: 15 mins

 Serves: 6

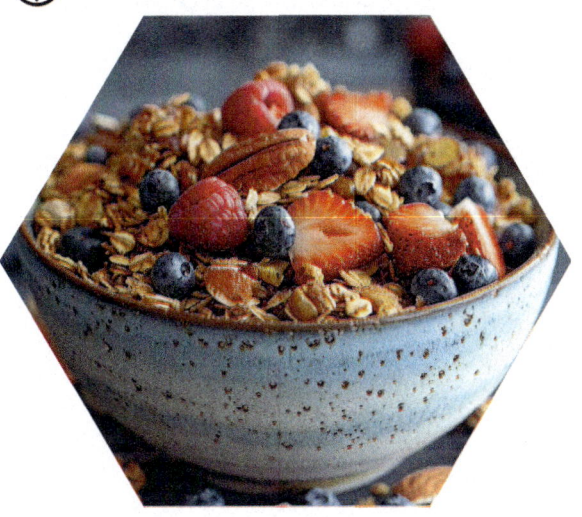

NUTRITION

- kcal: 298
- fat: 12g
- saturates: 4g
- carbs: 30g
- sugars: 10g
- fibre: 7g
- protein: 14g
- salt: 0.2g

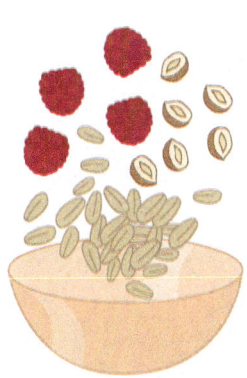

INGREDIENTS

- 50g (about 7) soft ready-to-eat dried apricots (we used Crazy Jack organic, because they are sulphur-free)
- ½ tbsp rapeseed oil
- 3 large eggs, whites only (see tip to use up the yolks)
- 200g porridge oats
- 1 tbsp cinnamon
- 1 tbsp vanilla extract
- 25g desiccated coconut
- 25g flaked almonds
- 25g pumpkin seeds
- 3 x 120g pots bio yogurt

3 peaches, to serve

DIRECTION

1. Preheat the oven to 180°C/160°C fan/gas 4 and line a large baking tray with parchment paper.

2. Blend apricots, oil, and egg whites until smooth. Stir in oats, cinnamon, and vanilla, then fold in coconut, almonds, and pumpkin seeds.

3. Pinch clusters of the mixture onto the lined tray, then bake for 15 minutes, toss, and bake for another 10 minutes until golden and crunchy

4. Cool completely on the tray, then store in an airtight jar. If following the Healthy Diet Plan, serve two portions over three days with yogurt and sliced peaches.

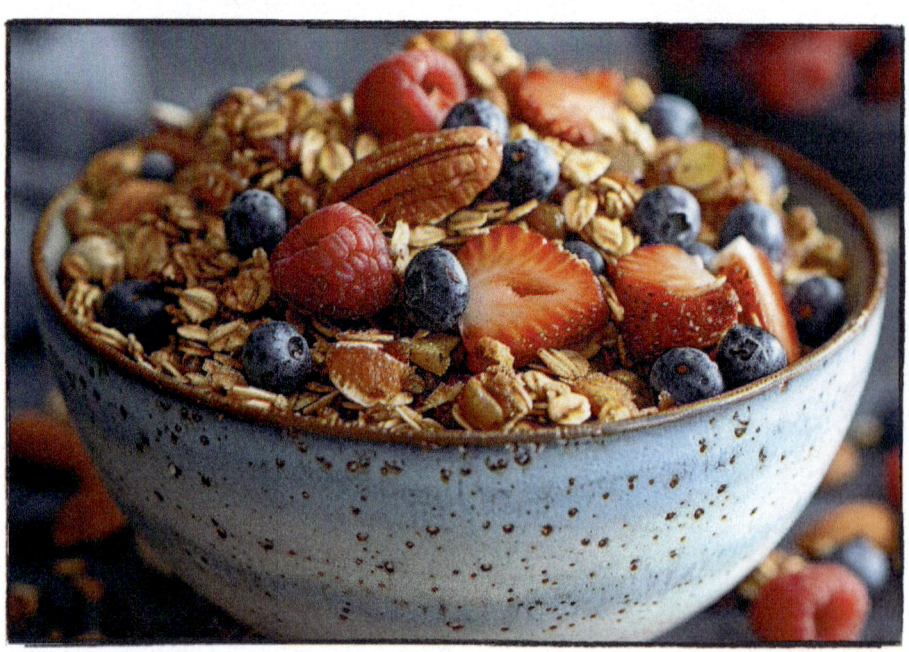

HEALTHY TUNA LETTUCE WRAPS

 Prep: 15 mins
Cook: 2 mins

 Serves: 2

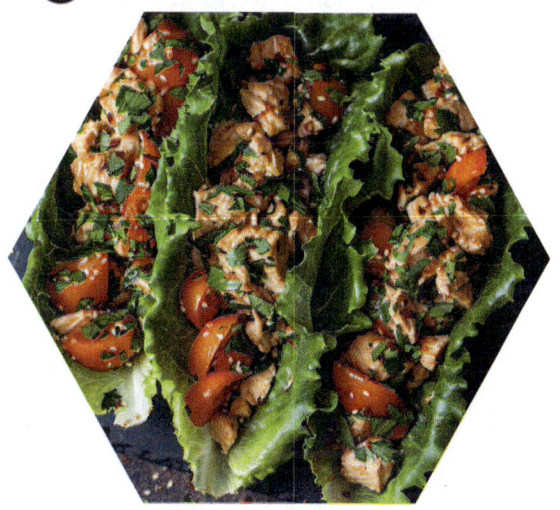

NUTRITION

- kcal: 361
- fat: 17g
- saturates: 3g
- carbs: 8g
- sugars: 7g
- fibre: 8g
- protein: 40g
- salt: 0.6g

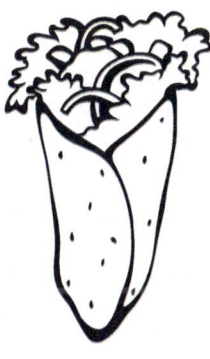

INGREDIENTS

- 2 drops rapeseed oil, for brushing
- 2 x 140g fresh tuna fillets, defrosted
- 1 ripe avocado
- ½ tsp English mustard powder
- 1 tsp cider vinegar
- 1 tbsp capers
- 8 romaine lettuce leaves
- 16 cherry tomatoes, preferably on the vine, halved

15

DIRECTION

1. Brush tuna with oil. Heat a non-stick pan and cook tuna for 1 minute on each side (or longer for thicker fillets). Transfer to a plate to rest.

2. Halve and pit avocado, then scoop flesh into a bowl. Add mustard powder and vinegar, mash until smooth like mayonnaise, then stir in capers. Spoon into two dishes and place on serving plates with lettuce leaves and tomatoes.

3. Slice tuna and arrange on plates. Spoon avocado mixture onto lettuce leaves, top with tuna, cherry tomatoes, and extra capers. Roll up to eat.

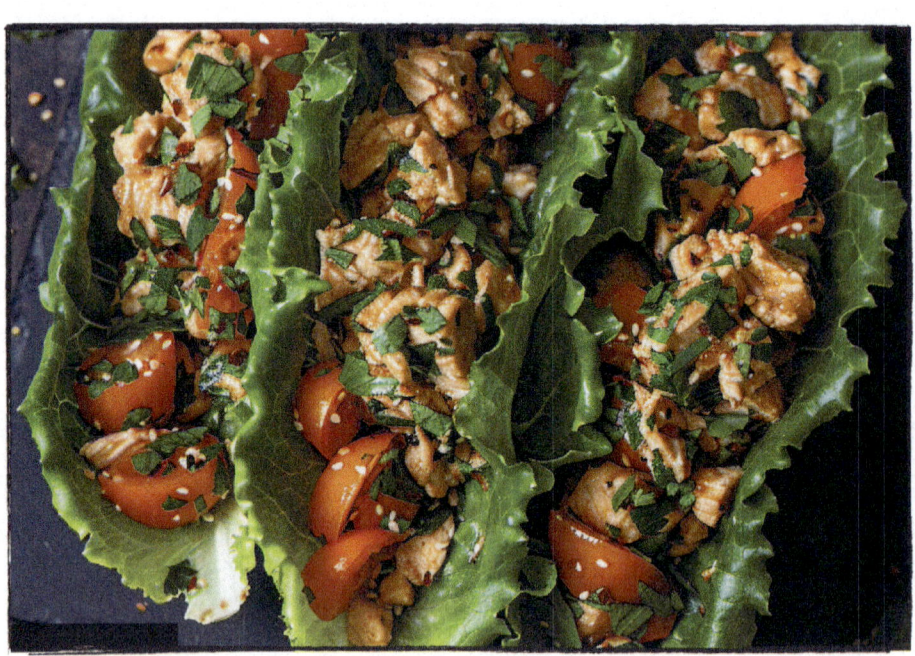

CHICKEN WITH CRUSHED HARISSA CHICKPEAS

Prep: 10 mins
Cook: 20 mins

 Serves: 2

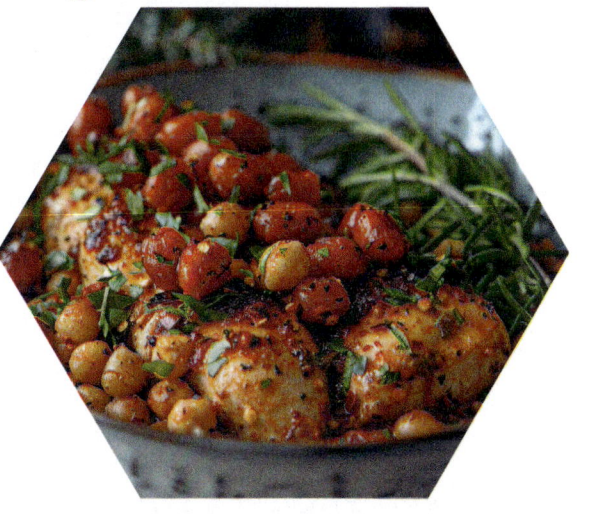

NUTRITION

- kcal: 366
- fat: 12g
- saturates: 2g
- carbs: 16g
- sugars: 6g
- fibre: 7g
- protein: 44g
- salt: 0.6g

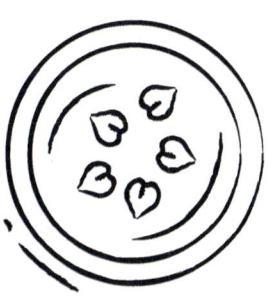

INGREDIENTS

- 2 tbsp rapeseed oil
- 1 onion, chopped
- 1 red pepper, finely sliced
- 1 yellow pepper, finely sliced
- 4 chicken breasts
- 1 tbsp za'atar
- 400g can chickpeas
- 1½ tbsp red harissa paste
- 150g baby spinach
- ½ small bunch of parsley, finely chopped
- lemon wedges, to serve

DIRECTION

1. Heat 1 tablespoon of oil in a frying pan over medium heat. Fry the onions and peppers for 7 minutes until softened and golden.

2. Meanwhile, place the chicken between two sheets of parchment paper and gently pound until about 2cm thick. Combine the remaining oil with za'atar, then rub it over the chicken. Season with salt and pepper.

3. Preheat the grill to high. Place the chicken on a foil-lined baking tray and grill for 3-4 minutes on each side, or until golden and cooked through.

4. Heat chickpeas in a pan with harissa paste and 2 tablespoons of water until warmed through, then mash roughly with a potato masher. Wilt the spinach in a pan with 1 tablespoon of water or in the microwave in a heatproof bowl. Combine the pepper and onion mixture, spinach, and parsley with the chickpeas. Serve with sliced chicken and lemon wedges for squeezing over.

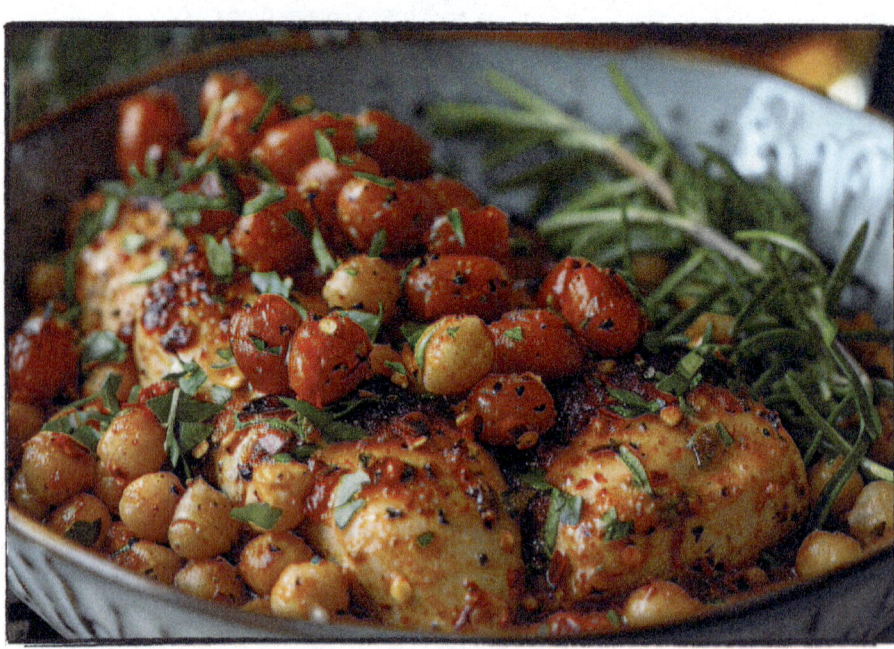

MEXICAN CHICKEN AND BEAN LIME SOUP

Prep: 10 mins
Cook: 20 mins

Serves: 2

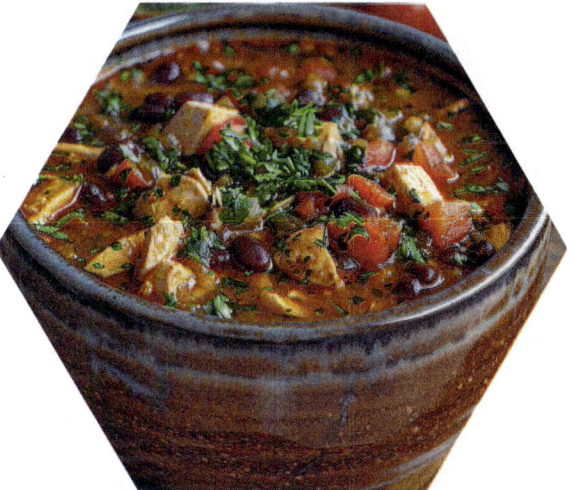

NUTRITION

- kcal: 38
- fat: 8g
- saturates: 1g
- carbs: 36g
- sugars: 17g
- fibre: 12g
- protein: 32g
- salt: 0.5g

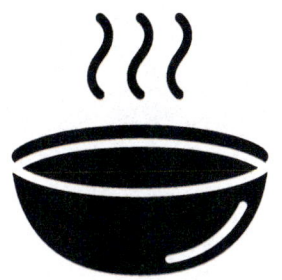

INGREDIENTS

- 2 tbsp rapeseed oil
- 1 onion, chopped
- 1 red pepper, finely sliced
- 1 yellow pepper, finely sliced
- 4 chicken breasts
- 1 tbsp za'atar
- 400g can chickpeas
- 1½ tbsp red harissa paste
- 150g baby spinach
- ½ small bunch of parsley, finely chopped
- lemon wedges, to serve

DIRECTION

1. Heat oil in a medium pan, add onion and pepper, and fry for 10 minutes, stirring frequently. Stir in garlic and spices, then add tomatoes and beans with their liquid, half a can of water, and bouillon powder. Simmer, covered, for 15 minutes.

2. Meanwhile, combine chicken, coriander, lime juice, and optional chili in a bowl, tossing well. Ladle soup into two bowls, top with chicken, and serve

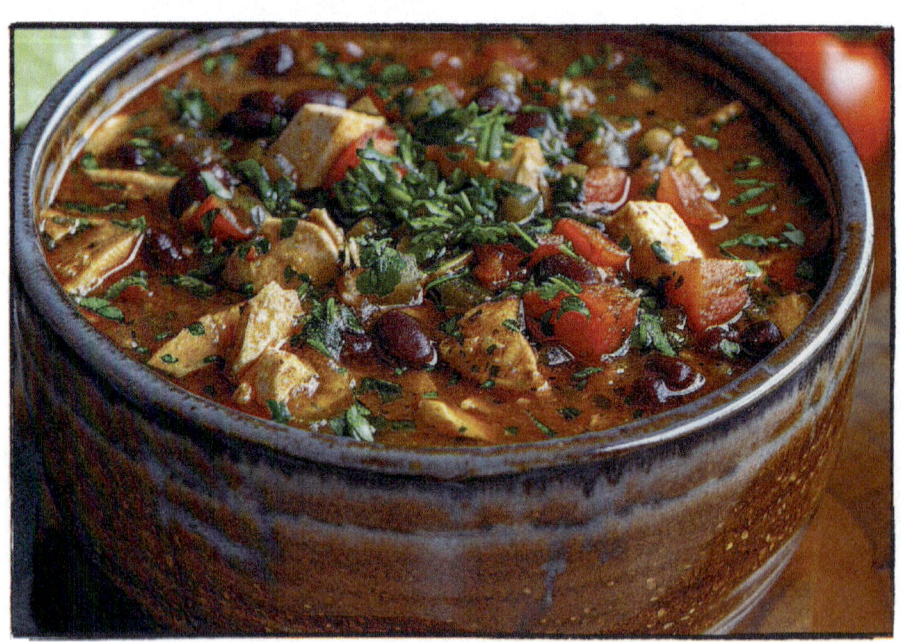

BARBECUE CHICKEN SALAD

 Prep: 20 mins
 Cook: 15 mins
Serves: 8

NUTRITION

- Calories: 301
- Fat: 14g
- Carbs: 32g
- Protein: 12g

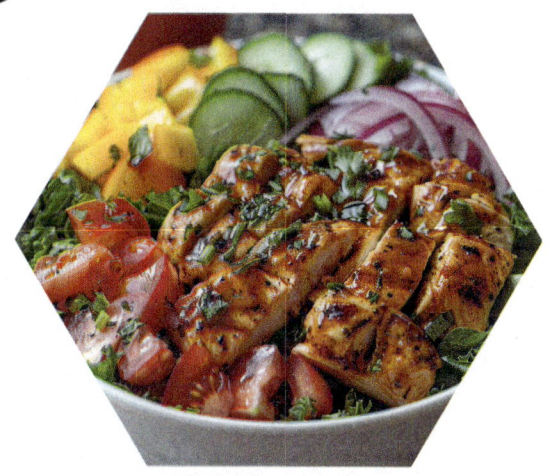

INGREDIENTS

- 2 skinless, boneless chicken breast halves
- 1 head red leaf lettuce, rinsed and torn
- 1 head green leaf lettuce, rinsed and torn
- 1 fresh tomato, chopped
- 1 bunch cilantro, chopped
- 1 (15.25 ounce) can whole kernel corn, drained
- 1 (15 ounce) can black beans, drained
- 1 (2.8 ounce) can French fried onions
- ½ cup ranch dressing
- ½ cup barbecue sauce

DIRECTION

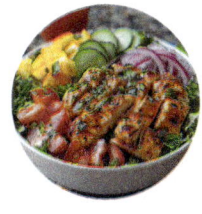

1. Preheat the grill for high heat and lightly oil the grate.
2. Cook chicken on the preheated grill until the juices run clear, about 6 minutes per side. An instant-read thermometer inserted into the center should read at least 165 degrees F (74 degrees C). Remove from heat, cool, and slice.
3. In a large bowl, mix lettuces, tomato, cilantro, corn, and black beans. Top with grilled chicken slices and French fried onions.
4. In a small bowl, mix ranch dressing and barbecue sauce together. Serve on the side as a dipping sauce or toss with the salad to coat.

FRESH FRUIT SALAD

 Prep: 15 mins
Cook: 15 mins

 Serves: 2

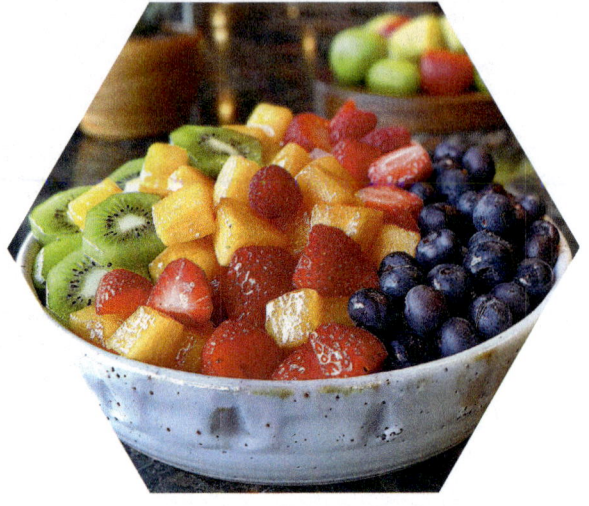

NUTRITION

- Calories: 156
- Fat: 1g
- Carbs: 38g
- Protein: 3g

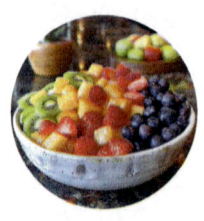

INGREDIENTS

- 1 small orange, peeled and diced
- ½ mango, diced
- ½ cup fresh blueberries
- ½ cup fresh strawberries, sliced
- ½ cup fresh raspberries
- ½ small banana, sliced
- 2 tablespoons plain yogurt
- 1 tablespoon maple syrup (Optional)
- 1 pinch white sugar

DIRECTION

1. Toss orange, mango, blueberries, strawberries, raspberries, and banana in a large bowl. Stir yogurt and syrup into the mixture to coat evenly. Sprinkle sugar over the salad; stir to serve.

BROCCOLI AND EGG PASTA SALAD WITH SUNFLOWER SEEDS

 Prep: 10 mins
Cook: 10 mins

 Serves: 2

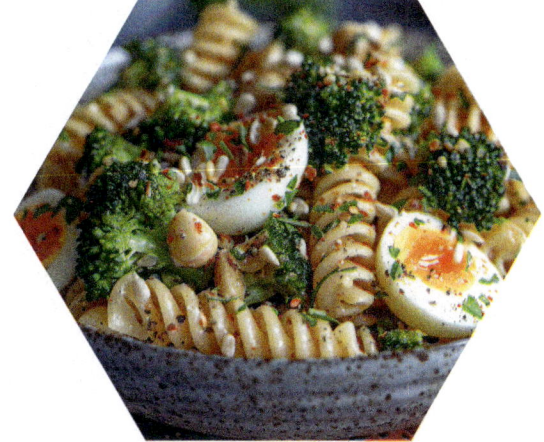

NUTRITION

- kcal: 436
- fat: 22g
- saturates: 4g
- carbs: 31g
- sugars: 5g
- fibre: 11g
- protein: 24g
- salt: 1.3g

INGREDIENTS

- 2 large eggs
- 75g wholewheat penne
- 160g broccoli florets
- 160g fine beans, trimmed and halved
- 1 tbsp white miso paste
- 1 tsp grated ginger
- 1 tbsp rapeseed oil
- 2 tbsp sunflower seeds

DIRECTION

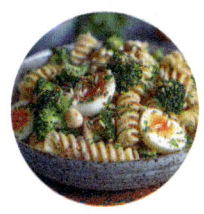

1. Hard-boil the eggs for 8 mins, then shell and halve. Meanwhile, boil the pasta for 5 mins, add the broccoli and beans, and cook 5 mins more or until everything is tender.
2. Drain, reserving the water, then tip the pasta and veg into a bowl and stir in the miso, ginger, oil and 4 tbsp pasta water. Serve topped with the eggs and seeds.

BLACK BEAN, CORN, AND QUINOA SALAD

Prep: 15 mins
Cook: 20 mins
 Serves: 6

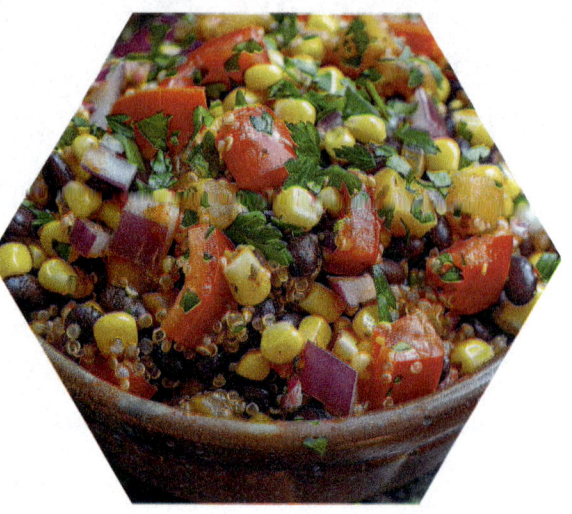

NUTRITION

- Calories: 250
- Fat: 7g
- Carbs: 38g
- Protein: 10g

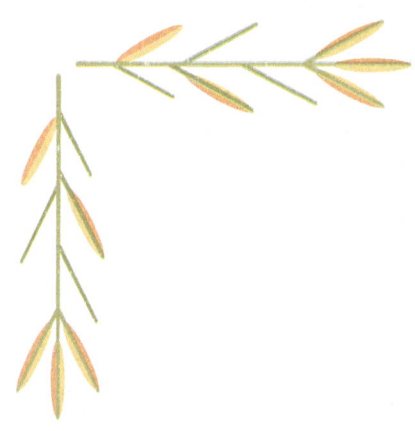

INGREDIENTS

- 2 cups chicken broth
- 1 cup uncooked quinoa
- 1 cup frozen corn
- 1 tablespoon lime juice
- 1 teaspoon red wine vinegar
- lime, zested
- ½ teaspoon ground cumin
- 2 tablespoons avocado oil
- 1 (15 ounce) can black beans, drained
- 1 small red bell pepper, seeded and chopped
- 1 small red onion, chopped
- ¼ cup chopped fresh cilantro
- salt and ground black pepper to taste

DIRECTION

1. Bring chicken broth to a boil in a 2-quart saucepan. Stir in quinoa. Reduce heat to low; simmer, covered, until broth is absorbed, 15 to 20 minutes. Remove from heat; stir in corn. Cover and let stand until corn is warmed through, about 5 minutes.

2. Whisk lime juice, red wine vinegar, lime zest, and cumin together in a large bowl. Whisk in avocado oil. Add black beans, red bell pepper, red onion, and cilantro. Season with salt and pepper. Stir in quinoa and corn.

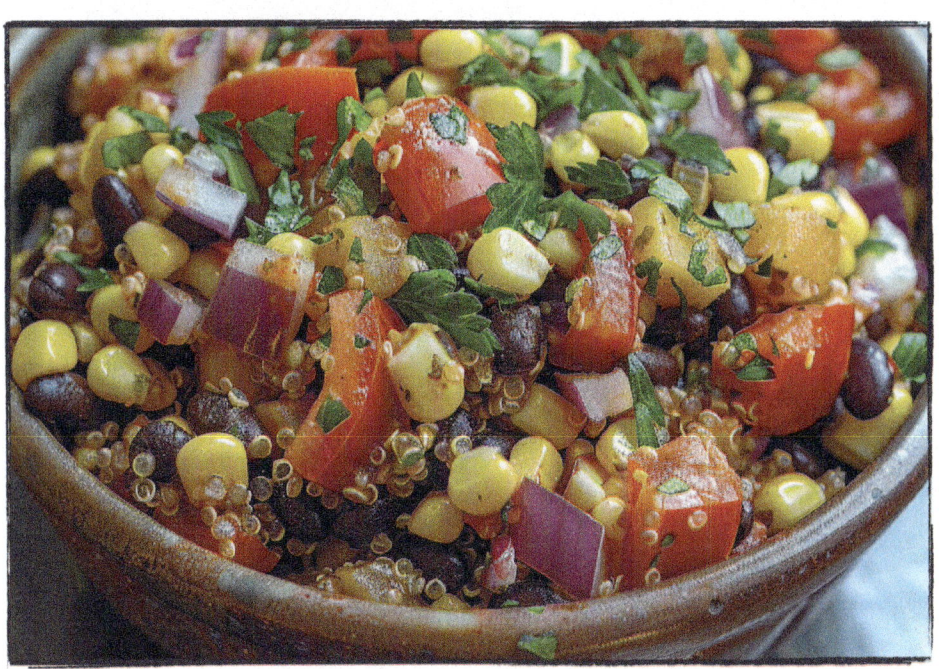

SOBA NOODLE SALAD WITH CHICKEN AND SESAME

 Prep: 20 mins
Cook: 7 mins

 Serves: 3

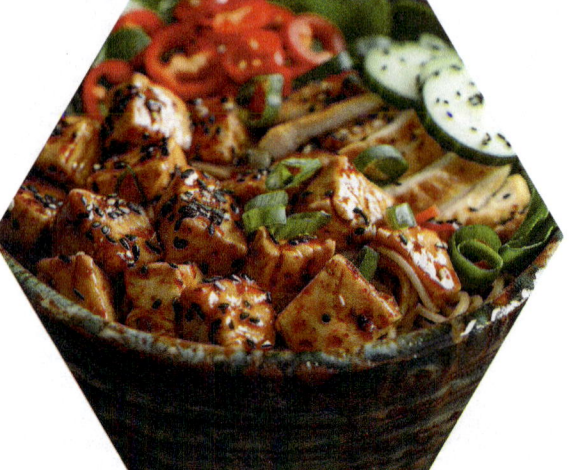

NUTRITION

- Calories: 340
- Fat: 15g
- Carbs: 38g
- Protein: 16g

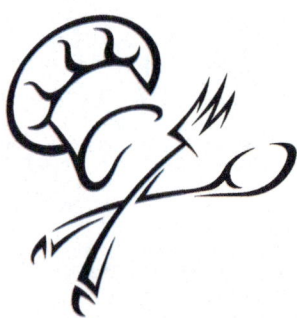

INGREDIENTS

- 2 tablespoons rice vinegar
- 1 tablespoon vegetable oil
- 1 tablespoon sesame oil
- 1 tablespoon brown sugar
- 1 tablespoon soy sauce
- 2 teaspoons minced fresh ginger root
- 4 ounces buckwheat soba noodles
- 2 teaspoons vegetable oil
- 1 boneless skinless chicken breast, cut into thin bite-size strips
- 1 teaspoon chopped garlic
- salt and ground black pepper to taste
- 1 rib celery, sliced (Optional)
- 1 carrot, sliced
- ½ red bell pepper, chopped
- ¼ cup chopped fresh cilantro
- 2 tablespoons chopped green onion
- 1 tablespoon sesame seeds

DIRECTION

1. Whisk rice vinegar, 1 tablespoon vegetable oil, sesame oil, brown sugar, soy sauce, and ginger together in a large bowl until dressing is combined.

2. Bring water to a boil in a large pot. Add soba noodles, stir, and return water to a boil. Boil noodles until tender, 4 to 5 minutes. Drain noodles in a colander under cold running water until cool, about 1 minute.

3. Heat 2 teaspoons vegetable oil in a skillet over medium heat. Cook chicken breast pieces until no longer pink in the center and the juices run clear, 2 to 4 minutes. Add garlic, salt, and pepper; stir until fragrant, about 1 minute more.

4. Toss soba noodles, chicken, celery, carrot, red pepper, cilantro, green onion, and sesame seeds together with dressing in large bowl.

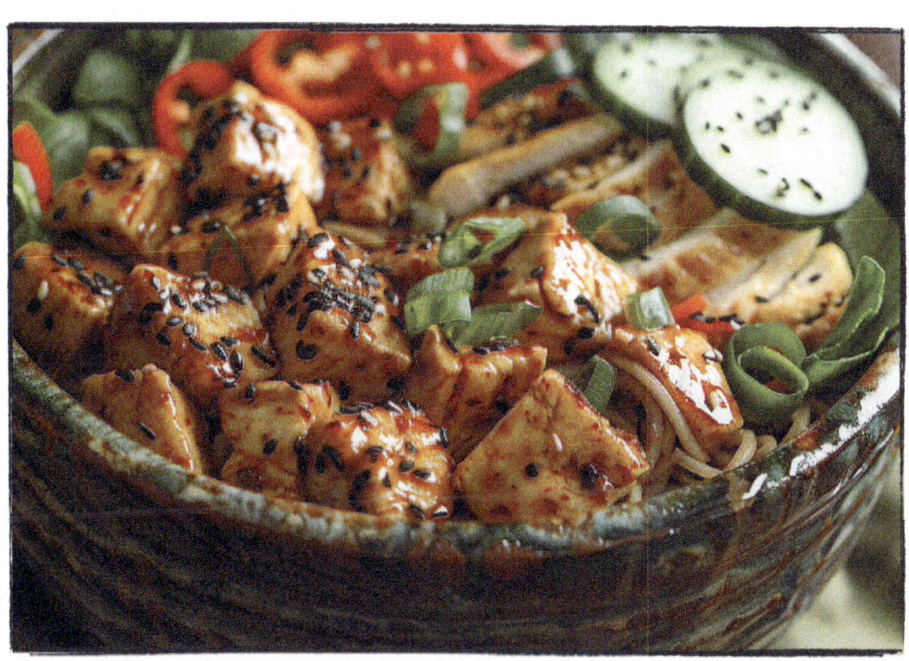

BLACK BEAN AND CORN SALAD

 Prep: 25 mins
 Serves: 6
Cook: 25 mins

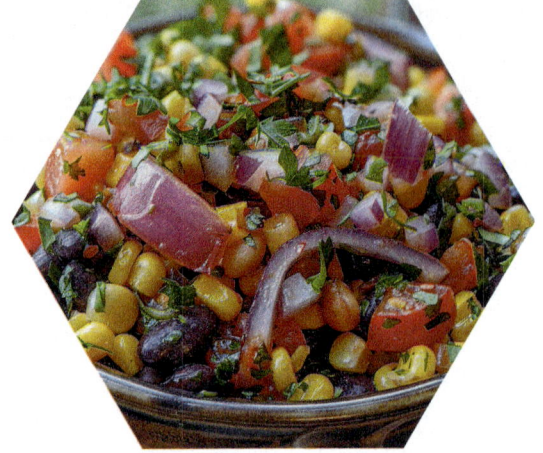

NUTRITION

- Calories: 391
- Fat: 25g
- Carbs: 35g
- Protein: 11g

INGREDIENTS

- ½ cup olive oil
- ⅓ cup fresh lime juice
- 1 clove garlic, minced
- 1 teaspoon salt
- ⅛ teaspoon ground cayenne pepper
- 2 (15 ounce) cans black beans, rinsed and drained
- 1 ½ cups frozen corn kernels
- 1 avocado - peeled, pitted and diced
- 1 red bell pepper, chopped
- 2 tomatoes, chopped
- 6 green onions, thinly sliced
- ½ cup chopped fresh cilantro

DIRECTION

1. Gather the ingredients.

2. Place olive oil, lime juice, garlic, salt, and cayenne pepper in a small jar. Close the lid tightly and shake the jar until the dressing is well combined.

3. Combine in a salad bowl beans, corn, avocado, bell pepper, tomatoes, green onions, and cilantro.

4. Shake dressing again, pour over salad, and toss to coat.

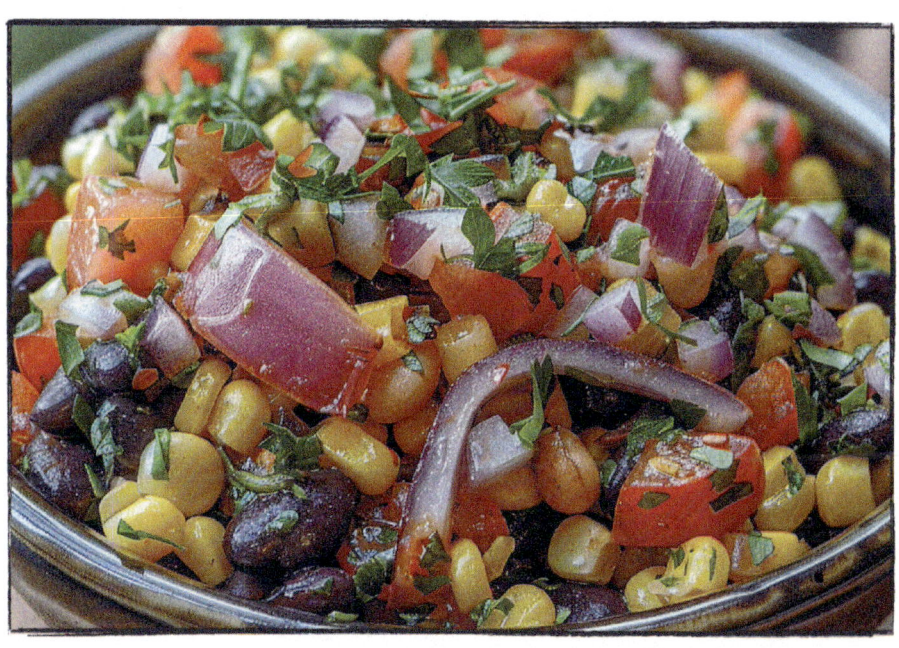

BEAKER'S VEGETABLE BARLEY SOUP

 Prep: 15 mins
 Cook: 1 hr 25 mins

 Serves: 8

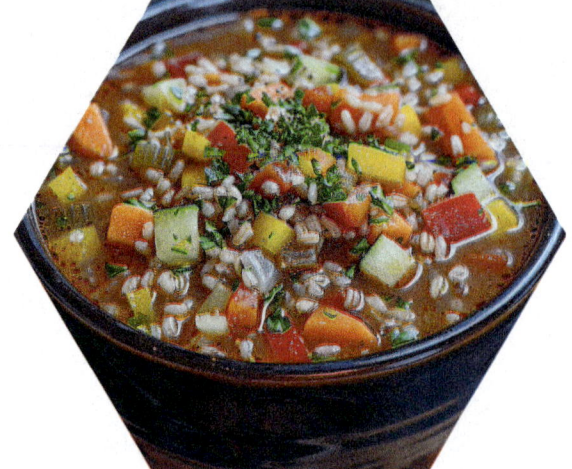

NUTRITION

- Calories: 313
- Fat: 1g
- Carbs: 79g
- Protein: 3g

INGREDIENTS

- 2 quarts vegetable broth
- 1 (15 ounce) can garbanzo beans, drained
- 1 (14.5 ounce) can diced tomatoes with juice
- 1 cup uncooked barley
- 2 large carrots, chopped
- 2 stalks celery, chopped
- 1 onion, chopped
- 1 zucchini, chopped
- 3 bay leaves
- 1 teaspoon garlic powder
- 1 teaspoon white sugar
- 1 teaspoon salt
- 1 teaspoon dried parsley
- 1 teaspoon curry powder
- 1 teaspoon paprika
- 1 teaspoon Worcestershire sauce
- ½ teaspoon ground black pepper

DIRECTION

 Pour broth into a large pot. Add beans, tomatoes with juice, barley, carrots, celery, onion, zucchini, and bay leaves. Season with garlic powder, sugar, salt, parsley, curry powder, paprika, Worcestershire sauce, and pepper. Bring to a boil, then reduce heat.

 Cover and simmer for 1 1/2 hours. Remove bay leaves before serving

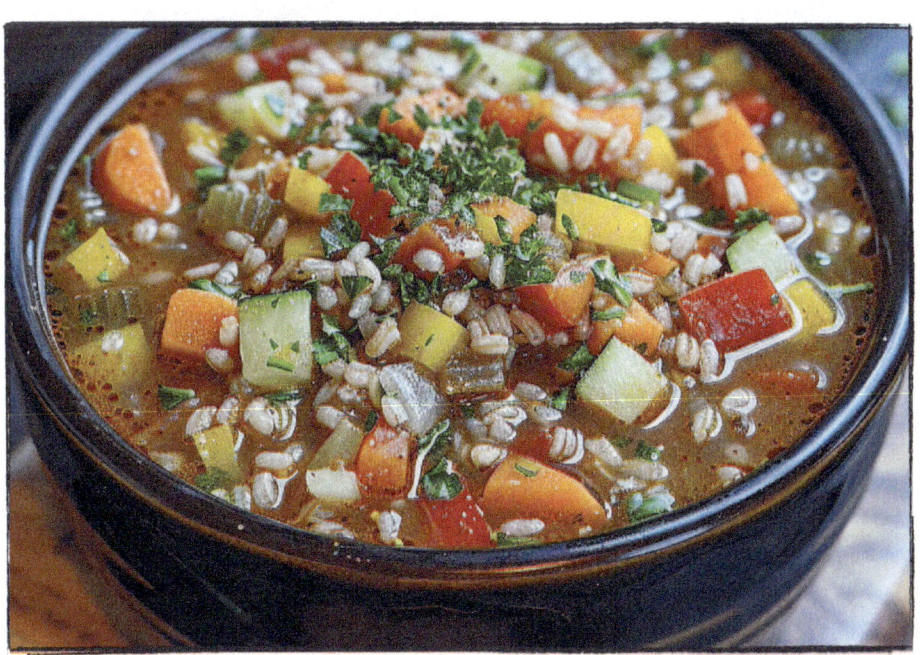

VEGAN UDON NOODLES SOUP WITH TOFU AND VEGETABLES

 Prep: 10 mins
 Cook: 30 mins

 Serves: 2

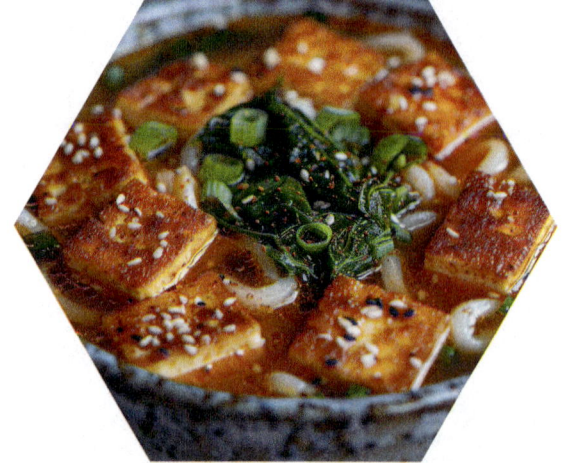

NUTRITION

- Calories: 271
- Fat: 9g
- Carbs: 38
- Protein: 10g

INGREDIENTS

- ½ (16 ounce) package tofu
- 6 ounces fresh udon noodles
- 1 tablespoon oil, or as needed
- 1 serrano pepper, minced, or to taste
- 1 teaspoon minced fresh ginger root
- 32 ounces vegetable broth
- 3 carrots, chopped
- ¼ cup chopped green onions
- ½ cup chopped bok choy
- 5 ounces shiitake mushrooms, chopped
- 1 teaspoon sesame oil
- 1 teaspoon soy sauce

DIRECTION

1. Wrap tofu in paper towels and place heavy books on top to dry out for 30 minutes.
2. Preheat oven to 400°F (200°C) and grease a baking sheet.
3. Chop pressed tofu into 1-inch cubes and place on the prepared baking sheet.
4. Bake in the preheated oven for 10 minutes, then turn tofu and bake for an additional 10 minutes until crispy.
5. While tofu bakes, bring a large pot of lightly salted water to a boil. Cook udon noodles according to package directions until tender yet firm, about 10 to 12 minutes. Drain.
6. Heat oil in a large pot over medium heat. Cook serrano pepper and ginger until softened, about 2 to 3 minutes.
7. Add vegetable broth, carrots, green onions, bok choy, shiitake mushrooms, sesame oil, soy sauce, and baked tofu. Bring to a boil, then reduce heat and simmer for 15 minutes, stirring occasionally.
8. Add cooked udon noodles and simmer for an additional 5 minutes.
9. Serve hot and enjoy!

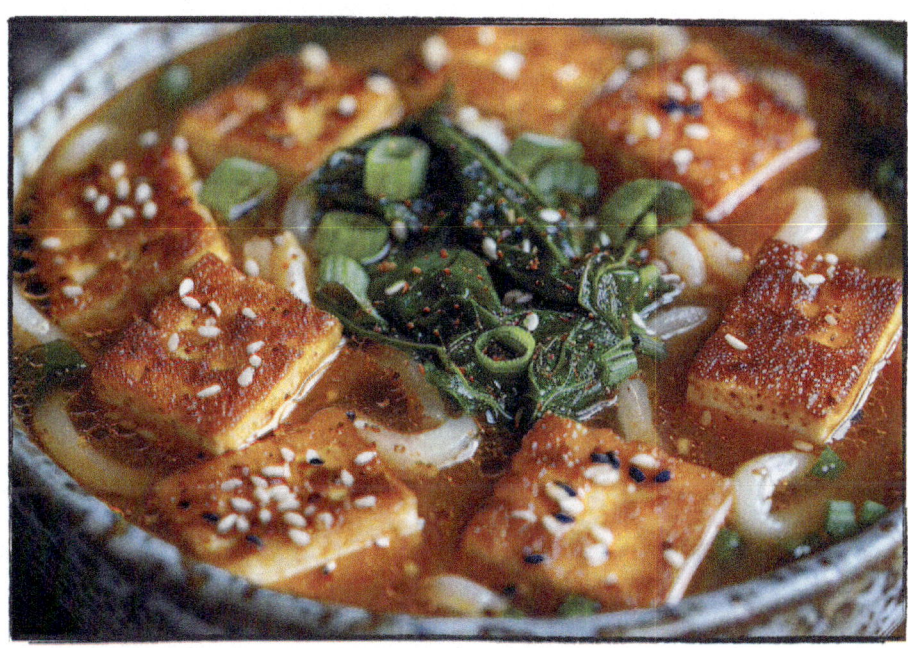

PUMPKIN SOUP

 Prep: 15 mins
Cook: 55 mins

 Serves: 6

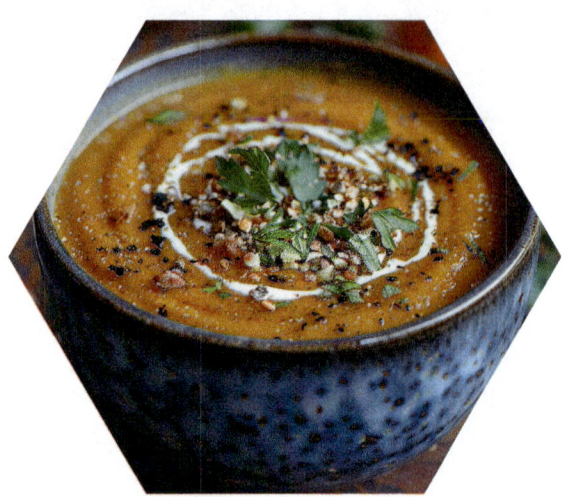

NUTRITION

- Calories: 223
- Fat: 12g
- Carbs: 25g
- Protein: 7g

INGREDIENTS

- 1 tablespoon olive oil
- 2 cups chopped yellow onion
- 10 whole black peppercorns
- 4 cloves garlic, minced
- 1 teaspoon chopped fresh thyme
- 3 cups pumpkin puree
- 4 cups chicken stock
- 3 tablespoons maple syrup (Optional)
- 3/4 teaspoon kosher salt
- 1/4 teaspoon ground nutmeg (Optional)
- 1/4 teaspoon ground cinnamon (Optional)
- ½ cup heavy whipping cream
- 2 tablespoons chopped fresh parsley

DIRECTION

1. Heat olive oil in a large pot over medium-high heat. Add onion and cook until browned and softened, about 10 minutes.
2. Add peppercorns, garlic, and thyme, and cook until fragrant and slightly browned, about 2 minutes.
3. Stir in pumpkin puree and cook until it darkens, about 5 minutes.
4. Add chicken stock, maple syrup, salt, nutmeg, and cinnamon. Bring to a simmer and cook, uncovered, until slightly reduced and flavors meld, about 30 minutes.
5. Transfer soup to a blender in batches and blend until smooth.
6. Return soup to the pot and stir in heavy cream. Cook until heated through, about 4 minutes.
7. Ladle soup into bowls and garnish with fresh parsley.

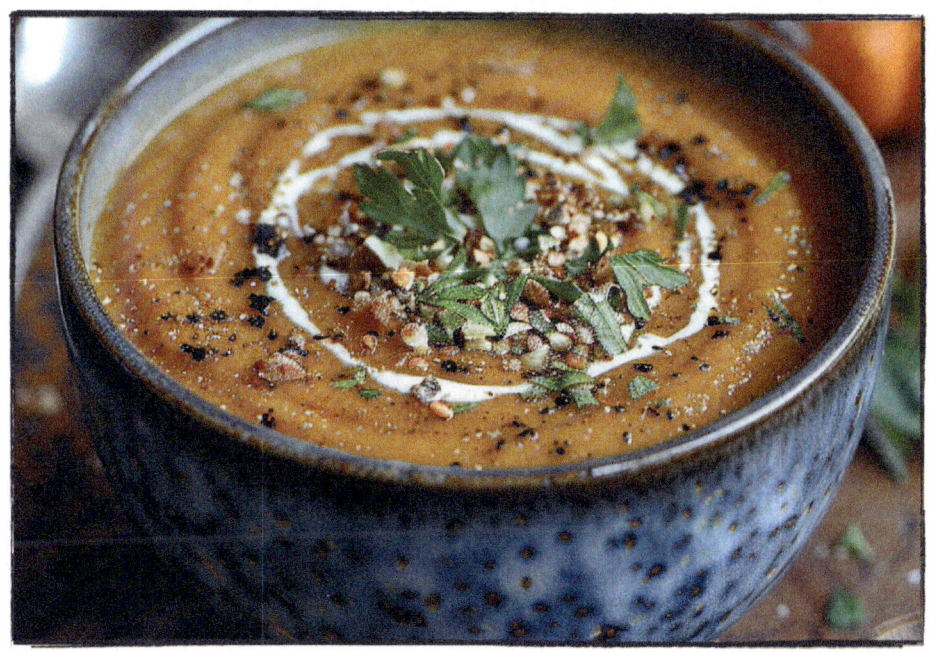

TOMATO BASIL SOUP

 Prep: 25 mins
 Cook: 30 mins

 Serves: 8

NUTRITION

- Calories: 270
- Fat: 25g
- Carbs: 10g
- Protein: 3g

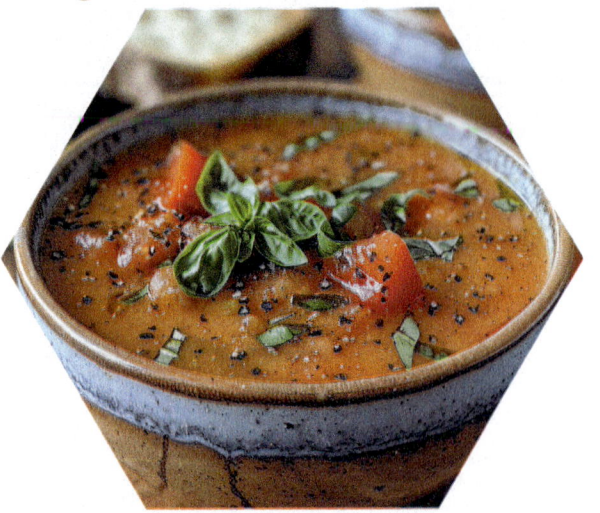

INGREDIENTS

- 6 tablespoons butter
- 1 onion, thinly sliced
- 15 baby carrots, thinly sliced
- 2 stalks celery, thinly sliced
- 3 cloves garlic, chopped
- 1 (28 ounce) can tomato sauce (such as Hunt's)
- 1 (8 ounce) can tomato sauce (such as Hunt's)
- 1 ¼ cups chicken broth
- 2 tablespoons chopped fresh basil
- 1 tablespoon chopped fresh oregano
- salt and ground black pepper to taste
- 1 ½ cups heavy whipping cream

DIRECTION

1 Melt butter in a large pot over medium-low heat; cook and stir onion, carrots, celery, and garlic until vegetables are tender, about 10 minutes.

2 Stir in both amounts of tomato sauce, chicken broth, basil, and oregano. Increase heat to medium and simmer until soup is reduced, 10 to 20 minutes.

3 Pour soup into a blender no more than half full. Cover and hold lid down; pulse a few times before leaving on to blend. Add cream. Continue to puree in batches until smooth, transferring creamy soup to another pot.

4 Heat soup over medium-high heat until hot, about 5 minutes more.

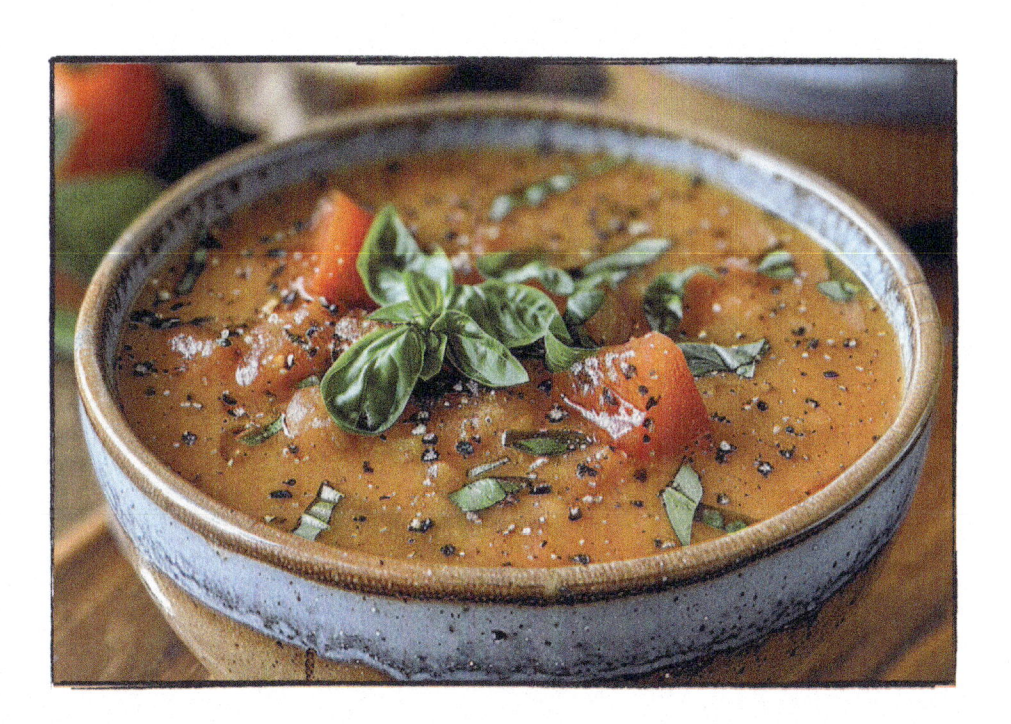

CHEF JOHN'S MISO SOUP

Prep: 20 mins
Cook: 20 mins
Serves: 4

NUTRITION

- Calories: 80
- Fat: 1g
- Carbs: 11g
- Protein: 7g

INGREDIENTS

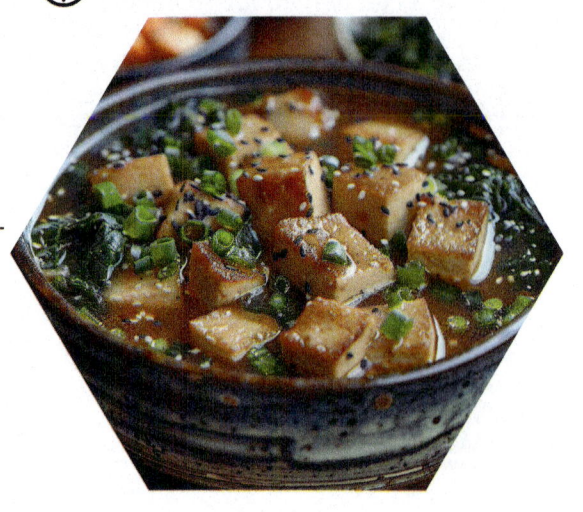

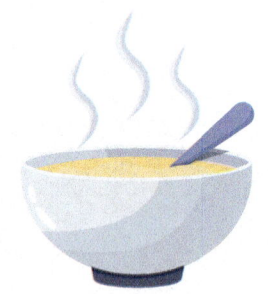

- Dashi:
- 6 cups cold water
- ½ ounce dried kombu (dried kelp)
- 2 cups lightly packed dried bonito flakes
- Miso Soup:
- 7 ounces silken tofu, drained and cut into 1/2-inch cubes
- 4 tablespoons white miso
- 2 tablespoons red miso
- dried wakame seaweed flakes
- shredded wakame or hijiki seaweed (soaked in water until soft) (Optional)
- 2 green onions, thinly sliced, plus more to garnish

DIRECTION

1. Gather all ingredients.
2. Pour cold water into a saucepan and add kombu, soaking for 30 minutes.
3. Set the pan on the stove over medium heat until the water just starts to simmer. Turn off the heat, remove the kombu, and discard it.
4. Turn the heat back on to medium-high and bring the liquid to a simmer. Stir in bonito flakes, then turn off the heat and let it sit for 10 minutes. Strain and reserve the liquid, known as "dashi."
5. Pour dashi into a saucepan over medium heat. Add pre-soaked, shredded seaweed, soy sauce, and green onions. Bring to a simmer, then reduce heat to low.
6. Place a small strainer over the pan and add miso pastes. Submerge the strainer halfway into the hot dashi, stirring slowly until all the miso dissolves and passes through into the soup.
7. Stir in tofu and continue cooking on low until tofu is heated through, about 2 minutes.
8. Taste and season with more soy sauce if needed.
9. Serve immediately with sliced green onions on top.

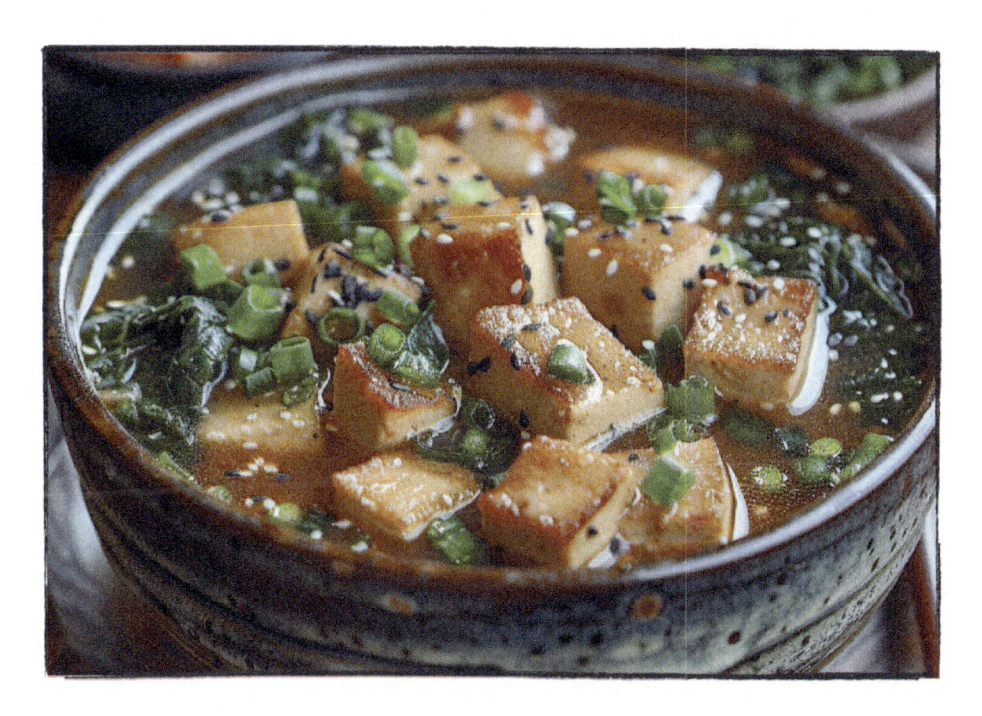

CHICKEN CORN BLACK BEAN SOUP

Prep: 15 mins
Cook: 20 mins
Serves: 6

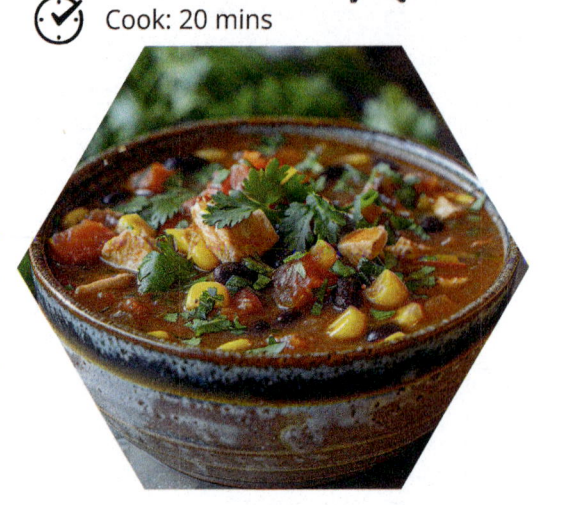

INGREDIENTS

- 1 cooked rotisserie chicken, shredded
- 32 ounces chicken broth
- 16 ounces restaurant-style salsa (such as Pace®)
- 1 (15.25 ounce) can sweet corn, drained
- 1 (15 ounce) can black beans, rinsed and drained
- 1 (11 ounce) can southwest-style corn, drained
- 1 (10.75 ounce) can condensed cream of chicken soup
- 1 (4 ounce) can mild, fire-roasted diced green chile peppers
- 2 ½ teaspoons ground cumin
- 1 teaspoon chili powder
- ½ teaspoon garlic powder
- ¼ teaspoon salt

NUTRITION

- kcal: 436
- fat: 22g
- saturates: 4g
- carbs: 31g
- sugars: 5g
- fibre: 11g
- protein: 24g
- salt: 1.3g

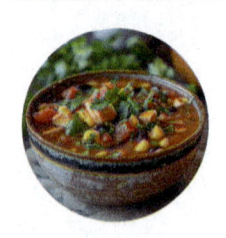

DIRECTION

1. Combine shredded chicken meat, chicken broth, salsa, sweet corn, black beans, southwest-style corn, condensed soup, diced green chiles, cumin, chili powder, garlic powder, and salt together in a large pot; bring to a boil.
2. Reduce heat to medium-low and simmer until heated through and flavors have blended, about 20 minutes.

LENTIL SOUP

Prep: 15 mins
Cook: 1 hr
Serves: 8

INGREDIENTS

- ¼ cup olive oil
- 1 onion, chopped
- 2 carrots, diced
- 2 stalks celery, chopped
- 2 cloves garlic, minced
- 1 bay leaf
- 1 teaspoon dried oregano
- 1 teaspoon dried basil
- 2 cups dry lentils
- 8 cups water
- 1 (14.5 ounce) can crushed tomatoes
- ½ cup spinach, rinsed and thinly sliced
- 2 tablespoons vinegar
- salt to taste
- ground black pepper to taste

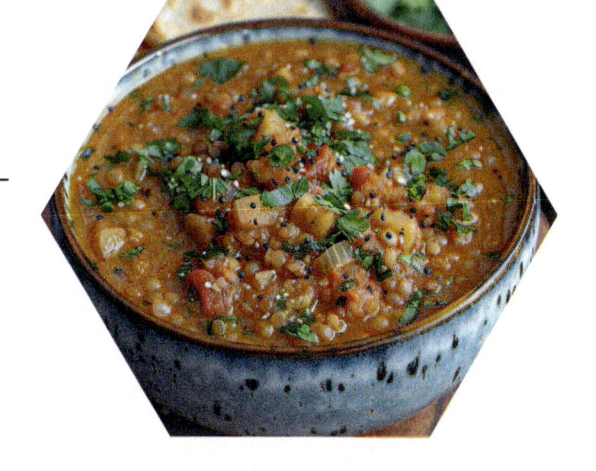

NUTRITION

- Calories: 349
- Fat: 10g
- Carbs: 48g
- Protein: 18g

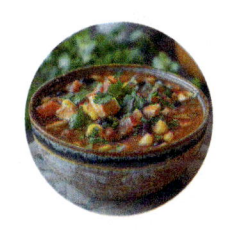

DIRECTION

1. Heat oil in a large soup pot over medium heat. Add onions, carrots, and celery; cook until onion is tender, about 3 to 5 minutes.
2. Stir in garlic, bay leaf, oregano, and basil; cook for 2 minutes.
3. Add lentils, water, and tomatoes. Bring to a boil, then reduce heat and simmer until lentils are tender, at least 1 hour.
4. When ready to serve, stir in spinach and cook until wilted.
5. Stir in vinegar and season with salt and pepper to taste.
6. Serve hot and enjoy!

CHICKEN WITH CRUSHED HARISSA CHICKPEAS

Prep: 10 mins
Cook: 20 mins
Serves: 2

NUTRITION

- kcal: 366
- fat: 12g
- saturates: 2g
- carbs: 16g
- sugars: 6g
- fibre: 7g
- protein: 44g
- salt: 0.6g

INGREDIENTS

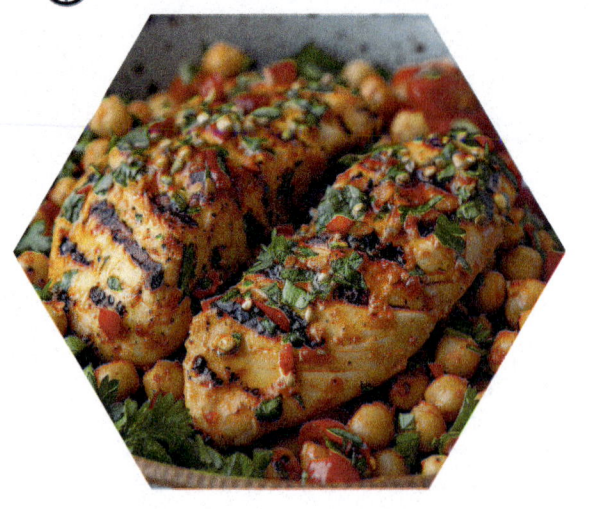

- 2 tbsp rapeseed oil
- 1 onion, chopped
- 1 red pepper, finely sliced
- 1 yellow pepper, finely sliced
- 4 chicken breasts
- 1 tbsp za'atar
- 400g can chickpeas
- 1½ tbsp red harissa paste
- 150g baby spinach
- ½ small bunch of parsley, finely chopped
- lemon wedges, to serve

DIRECTION

1 Heat 1 tablespoon of oil in a frying pan over medium heat. Fry the onions and peppers for 7 minutes until softened and golden.

2 Meanwhile, place the chicken between two sheets of parchment paper and gently pound until about 2cm thick. Combine the remaining oil with za'atar, then rub it over the chicken. Season with salt and pepper.

3 Combine in a salad bowl beans, corn, avocado, bell pepper, tomatoes, green onions, and cilantro.

4 Heat chickpeas in a pan with harissa paste and 2 tablespoons of water until warmed through, then mash roughly with a potato masher. Wilt the spinach in a pan with 1 tablespoon of water or in the microwave in a heatproof bowl. Combine the pepper and onion mixture, spinach, and parsley with the chickpeas. Serve with sliced chicken and lemon wedges for squeezing over.

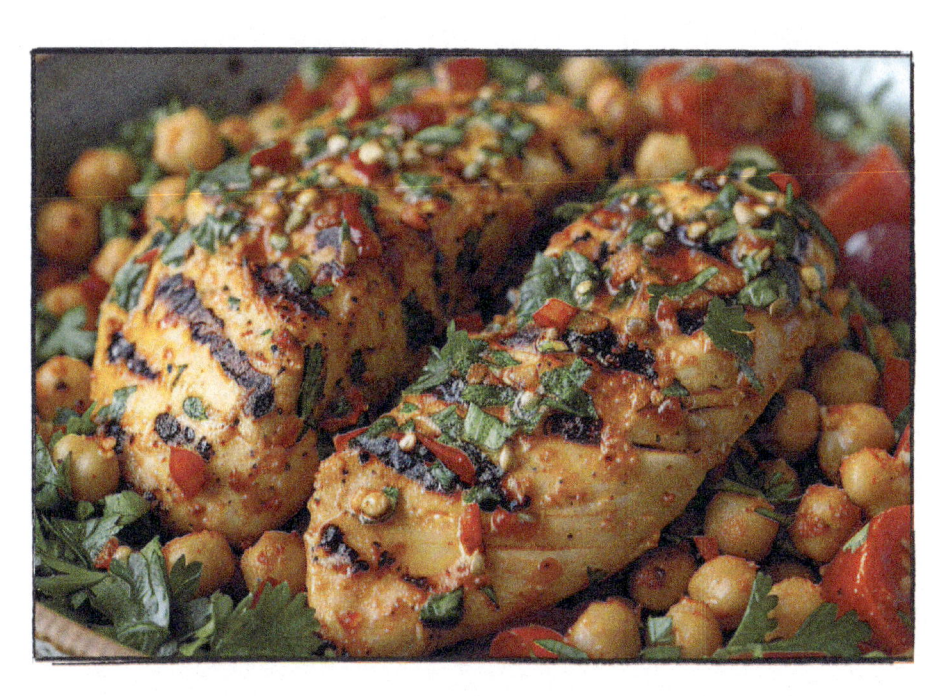

CURRIED COD

Prep: 5 mins
Cook: 15 mins
Serves: 6

NUTRITION

- Calories: 227
- Fat: 8g
- Carbs: 11g
- Protein: 24g

INGREDIENTS

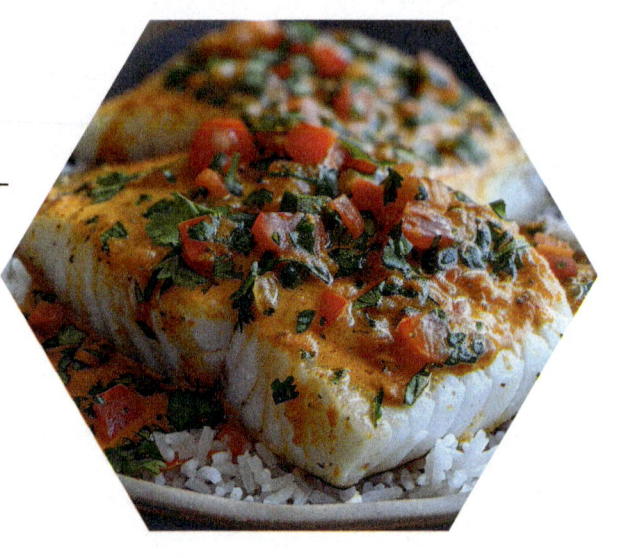

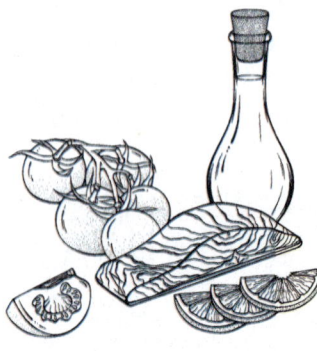

- 2 tablespoons vegetable oil
- 1 medium onion, chopped
- 1 teaspoon garlic paste
- 1 teaspoon ginger paste
- 2 teaspoons cumin
- 2 teaspoons coriander
- 1 teaspoon cardamom
- ½ teaspoon turmeric
- ½ teaspoon salt
- 2 fresh jalapeno peppers, seeded and diced
- .23999999463558 cup chopped cilantro
- 1 tablespoon lemon juice
- 1 (28 ounce) can diced tomatoes with juice
- 1 pound cod fillets, cut into chunks

DIRECTION

1 Heat the oil in a skillet over medium heat. Place onion in the skillet. Reduce heat to low, and cook, stirring often, 15 minutes, or until soft and brown.

2 Mix the garlic paste and ginger paste into the skillet. Cook 1 minute. Mix in cumin, coriander, cardamom, turmeric, and salt. Stir in the jalapeno, cilantro, lemon juice, and tomatoes with juice, scraping up any brown bits from the bottom of the skillet. Bring to a boil. Reduce heat to low, cover, and simmer 20 minutes. If you like, the sauce may be set aside for a few hours at this point to allow the flavors to blend.

3 Combine in a salad bowl beans, corn, avocado, bell pepper, tomatoes, green onions, and cilantro.

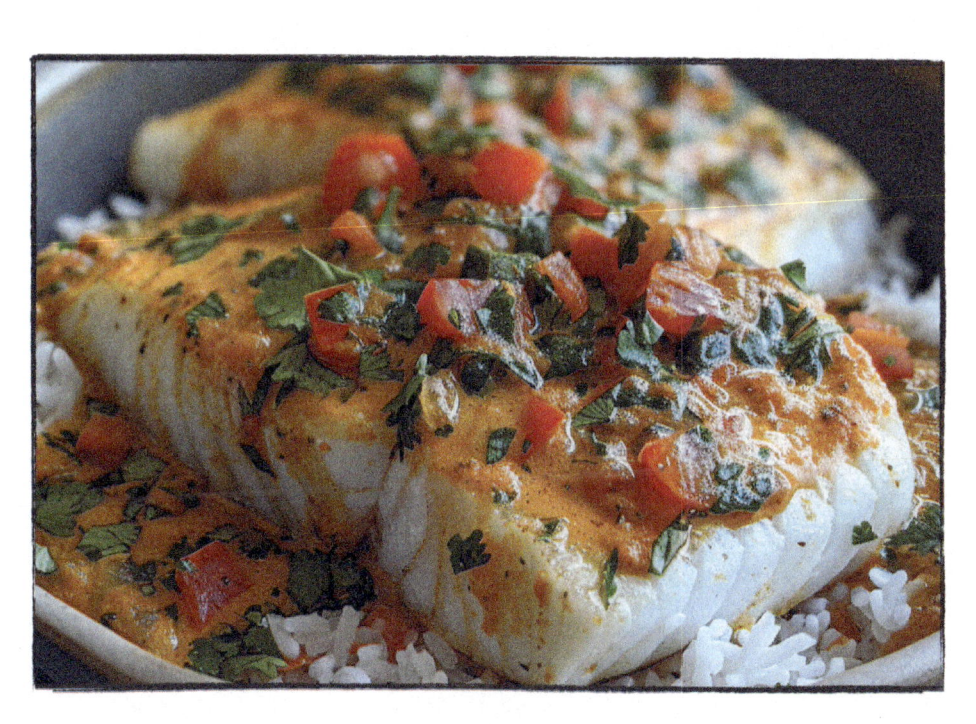

LEMON HERB GRILLED SALMON

Prep: 15 mins
Cook: 15 mins
Serves: 6

INGREDIENTS

- ½ cup olive oil
- ¼ cup lemon juice
- 4 green onions, thinly sliced
- 1 tablespoon chopped fresh parsley
- 1 teaspoon chopped fresh rosemary
- 1 teaspoon chopped fresh thyme
- ½ teaspoon salt
- ⅛ teaspoon black pepper
- ⅛ teaspoon garlic powder
- 3 pounds salmon fillets

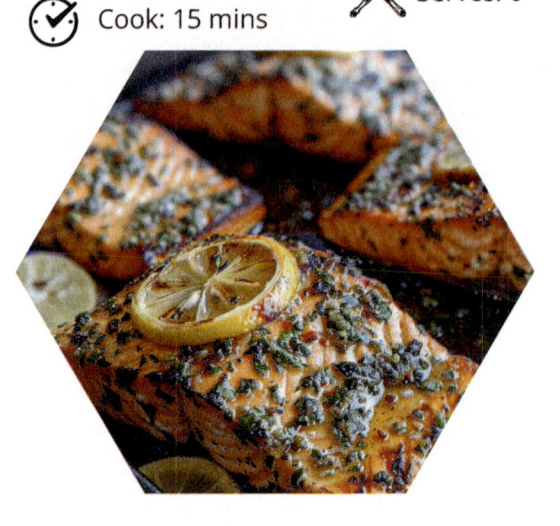

NUTRITION

- Calories: 301
- Fat: 14g
- Carbs: 32g
- Protein: 12g

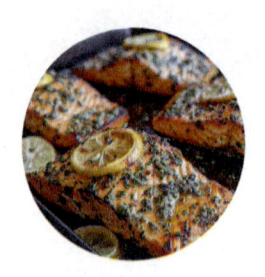

DIRECTION

1. Combine olive oil, lemon juice, green onions, parsley, rosemary, thyme, salt, black pepper, and garlic powder in a small bowl; reserve 1/4 cup for basting.
2. Place salmon fillets in a shallow dish and pour remaining marinade on top. Cover and refrigerate for 30 minutes.
3. Preheat the grill for medium heat and lightly oil the grate.
4. Remove fillets from the refrigerator; discard marinade. Place fillets on the preheated grill skin-side down. Cook, basting occasionally with reserved marinade, until fish flakes easily with a fork, 15 to 20 minutes.

SHRIMP AND QUINOA

Prep: 15 mins
Cook: 40 mins

Serves: 4

NUTRITION

- Calories: 458
- Fat: 18g
- Carbs: 44g
- Protein: 31g

INGREDIENTS

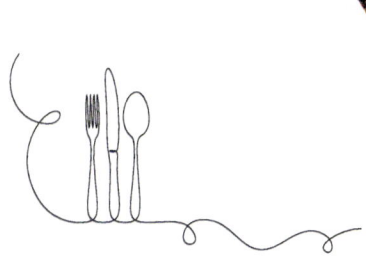

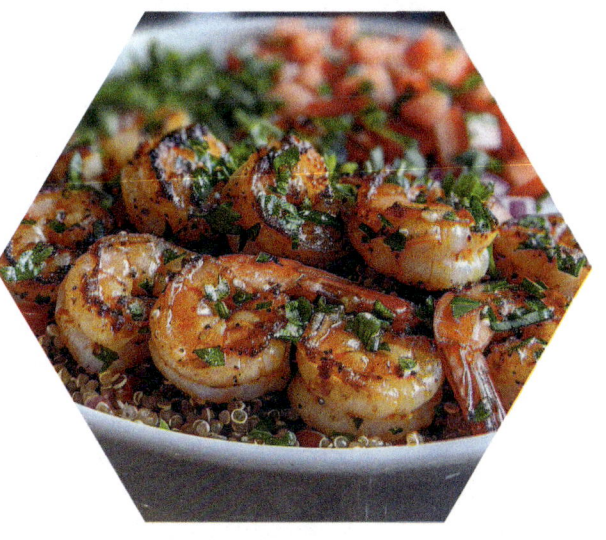

- 1 ½ cups water
- 1 cup uncooked quinoa
- 2 tablespoons olive oil
- 1 red onion, chopped
- ½ green bell pepper, chopped
- ½ cup sliced fresh mushrooms
- 6 fresh asparagus spears, trimmed and chopped
- ¼ cup golden raisins
- 1 tablespoon minced fresh ginger root
- salt and pepper to taste
- 1 pound medium shrimp - peeled and deveined
- 1 lime, juiced
- 2 tablespoons olive oil
- ½ cup chopped Italian flat leaf parsley

DIRECTION

1 In a large pot, bring the water to a boil, and stir in the quinoa. Cover, reduce heat to low, and simmer 15 minutes. Remove from heat, and set aside 10 minutes, or until all liquid has been absorbed.

2 Heat 2 tablespoons olive oil in a skillet over medium heat, and saute the onion and green bell pepper until tender. Mix in the mushrooms, asparagus, raisins, and ginger, and continue cooking until asparagus is tender. Season with salt and pepper. Mix in the shrimp, and cook 5 minutes, or until opaque.

3 In a large bowl, mix the quinoa with the lime juice and remaining 2 tablespoons olive oil. Toss with the skillet mixture and parsley to serve.

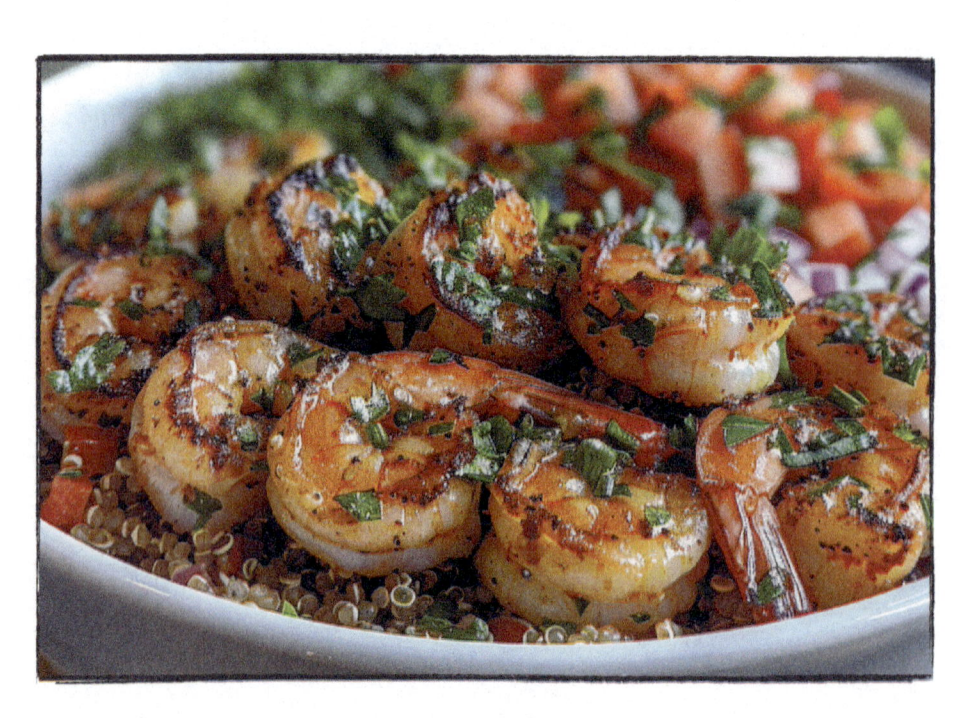

SHRIMP AND BROCCOLI STIR-FRY

Prep: 30 mins
Cook: 15 mins
Serves: 4

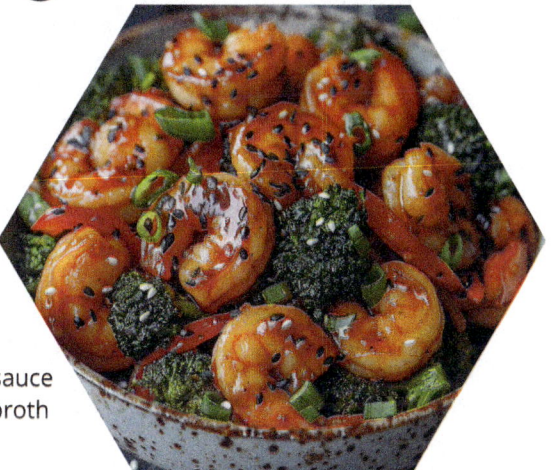

INGREDIENTS

Sauce:
- 1 cup reduced-sodium soy sauce
- ½ cup low-sodium chicken broth
- 2 tablespoons orange juice
- 1 tablespoon fish sauce
- 1 tablespoon rice vinegar
- 1 teaspoon garlic powder
- 1 teaspoon ginger powder
- ½ teaspoon Sriracha sauce, or to taste
- ½ teaspoon sesame oil

Stir-Fry:
- 3 tablespoons peanut oil, or more as needed
- 1 tablespoon thinly sliced garlic
- 1 tablespoon thinly sliced ginger
- 1 (12 ounce) bag broccoli - cut into florets, stems peeled and sliced 1/4 inch thick
- ⅔ cup onion, cut into long slices
- ⅔ cup red bell pepper, cut into long thin strips
- ⅔ cup carrots, cut diagonally into thin slices
- ⅔ cup fresh snow peas, trimmed
- 1 pound large shrimp (21-25 per pound), peeled and deveined

NUTRITION

- Calories: 401
- Fat: 14g
- Carbs: 40g
- Protein: 30g

DIRECTION

1. Combine soy sauce, chicken broth, orange juice, fish sauce, rice vinegar, garlic powder, ginger powder, Sriracha sauce, and sesame oil in a large jar with a lid. Close and shake until sauce is well combined. Set aside.
2. Heat peanut oil in a large, non-stick skillet or wok over medium-high heat. Add garlic and ginger and cook, stirring, until garlic and ginger are lightly browned, 1 to 2 minutes. Remove from the hot oil with a slotted spoon and discard.
3. Add broccoli, onion, bell pepper, carrots, and snow peas to the seasoned oil and cook, stirring quickly, until vegetables are tender-crisp and brightly colored, 3 to 4 minutes. Remove to a plate and keep warm.
4. Add shrimp to the hot skillet and cook for 90 seconds. Turn shrimp and continue cooking on the other side until they are bright pink on the outside, the meat is opaque, and shrimp begin to curl into a "C" shape, about 90 seconds longer.
5. Add stir-fried vegetables back to the skillet, and pour in sauce.
6. Mix together cornstarch and water in a small bowl and add to the sauce, stirring to remove any lumps. Keep stirring quickly, until thickener is incorporated into the entire dish. Bring to a boil, stirring constantly, then remove from heat.
7. Serve with hot, fluffy rice, and garnish with sesame seeds.

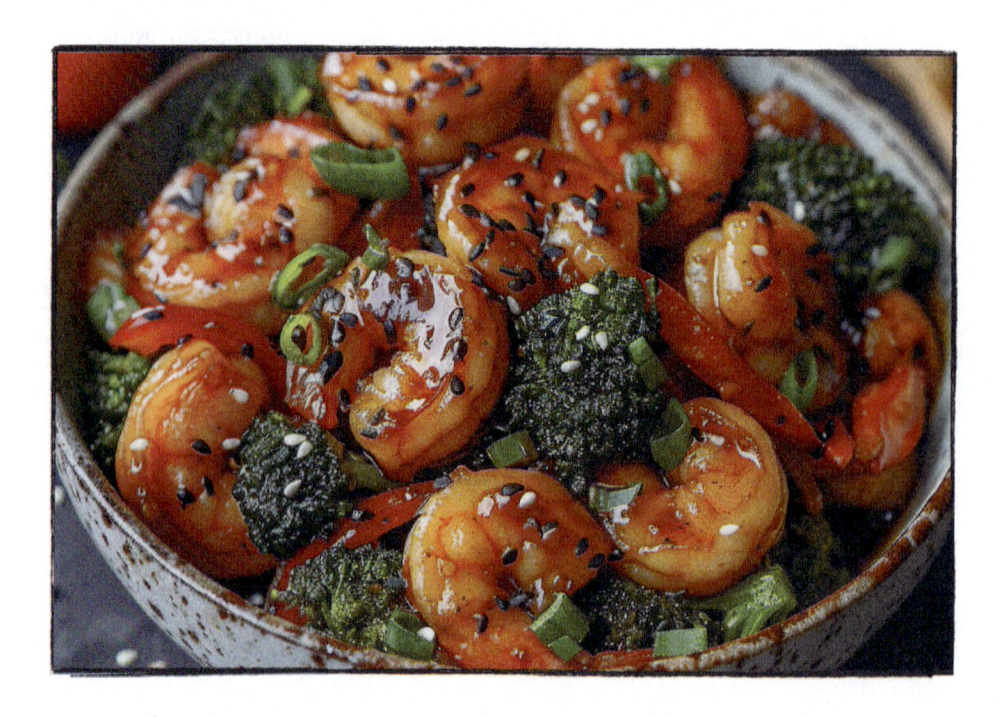

GRILLED PORK TENDERLOIN

Prep: 10 mins
Cook: 45 mins

Serves: 8

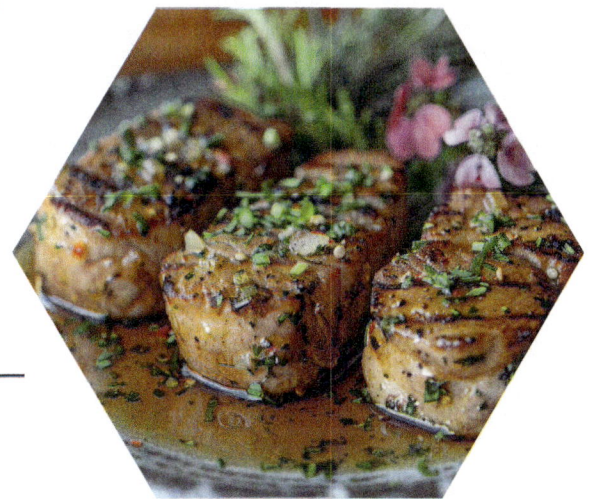

NUTRITION

- Calories: 185
- Fat: 4g
- Carbs: 12g
- Protein: 24g

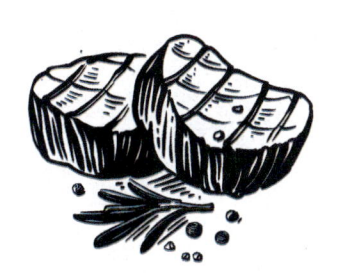

INGREDIENTS

- 2 (1 pound) pork tenderloins
- 1 teaspoon garlic powder
- 1 teaspoon salt
- 1 teaspoon ground black pepper
- 1 cup barbecue sauce, divided

DIRECTION

1. Gather all ingredients.
2. Preheat an outdoor grill for medium, indirect heat and lightly oil the grate.
3. Season tenderloins with garlic powder, salt, and pepper.
4. Place 1/2 of the barbecue sauce into a small bowl for basting; set aside remaining barbecue sauce for serving.
5. Cook pork on the preheated grill over indirect heat for 30 minutes.
6. Brush pork with barbecue sauce, turn, and brush again, using all sauce in the small bowl.
7. Continue cooking until an instant-read thermometer inserted into the center reads 145°F (63°C), about 15 more minutes.
8. Let pork rest for 10 minutes.
9. Slice pork and serve with reserved barbecue sauce.

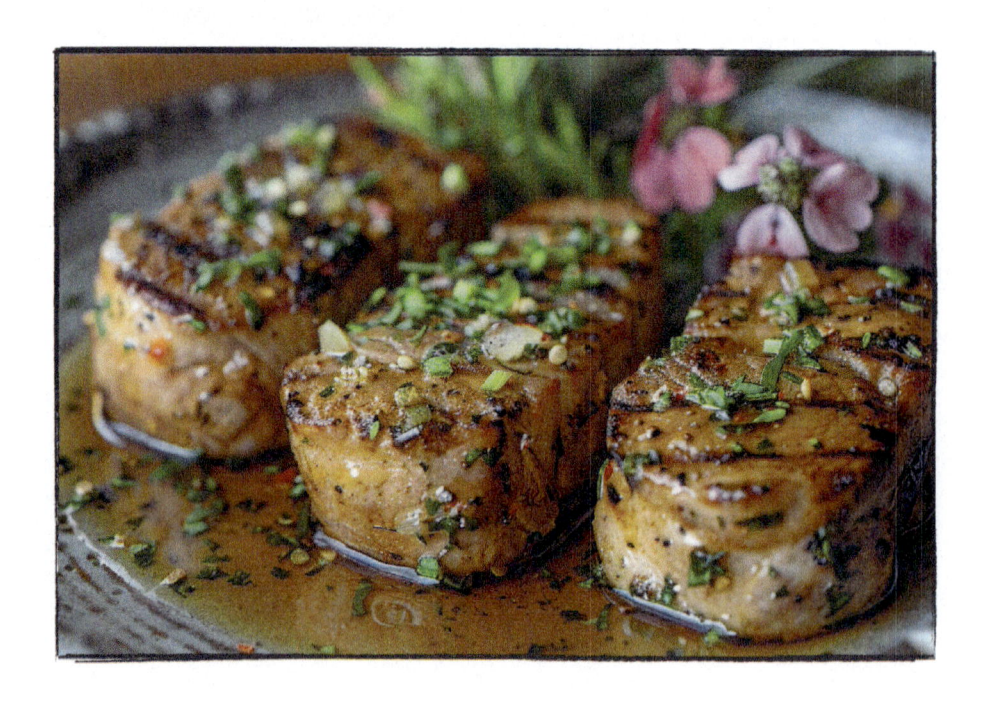

STIR-FRIED CHICKEN WITH TOFU AND MIXED VEGETABLES

Prep: 15 mins
Cook: 15 mins
Serves: 6

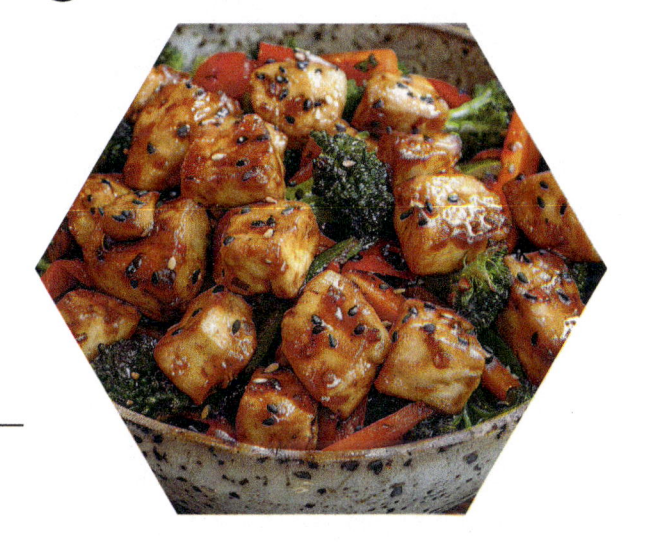

NUTRITION

- Calories: 172
- Fat: 6g
- Carbs: 12g
- Protein: 18g

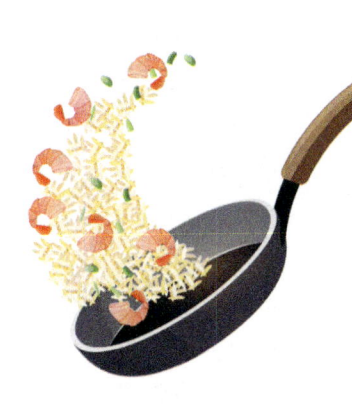

INGREDIENTS

- 3 tablespoons light soy sauce
- 1 teaspoon white sugar
- 1 tablespoon cornstarch
- 3 tablespoons Chinese rice wine
- 1 medium green onion, diced
- 2 skinless, boneless chicken breast halves - cut into bite-size pieces
- 3 cloves garlic, chopped
- 1 yellow onion, thinly sliced
- 2 green bell peppers, thinly sliced
- 1 (12 ounce) package firm tofu, drained and cubed
- ½ cup water
- 2 tablespoons oyster sauce
- 1 ½ tablespoons chili paste with garlic

DIRECTION

1 In a medium bowl, mix the soy sauce, sugar, cornstarch, and rice wine. Place the green onion and chicken in the mixture. Allow to marinate at least 15 minutes.

2 In a wok over medium-high heat, cook and stir the chicken with the marinade mixture about 5 minutes until almost done. Toss in the garlic, onion, and peppers. Continue to cook and stir 5 minutes, or until vegetables are crisp but tender and chicken is no longer pink and juices run clear.

3 Mix the tofu, water, oyster sauce, and chili paste into the wok. Cook and stir until heated through.

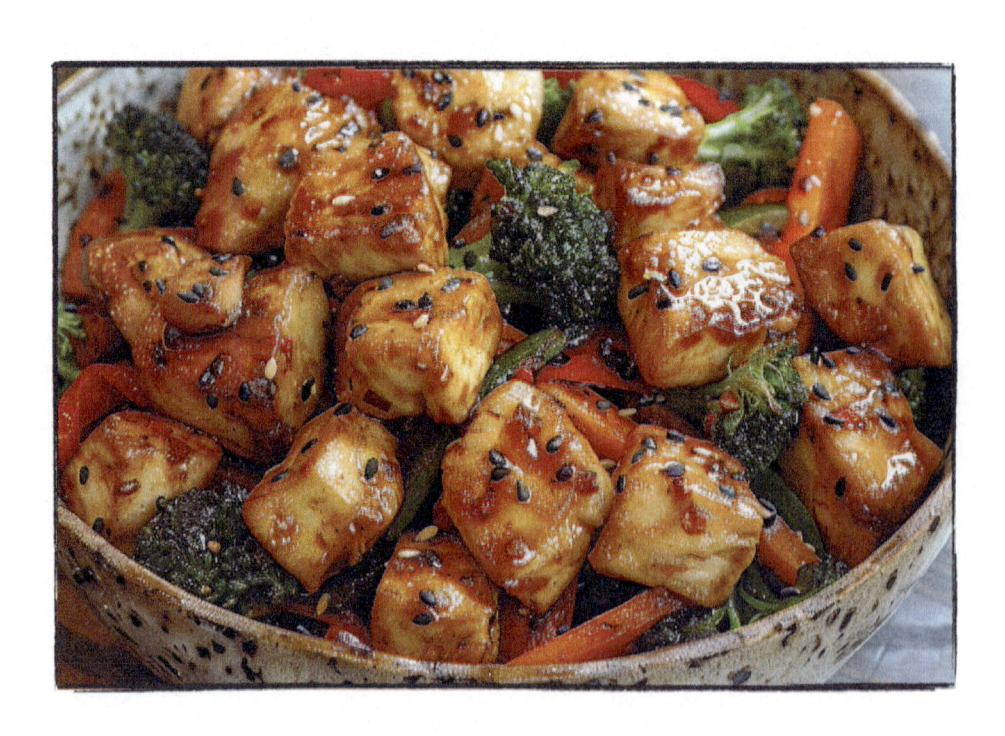

SIMPLE TURKEY CHILI

Prep: 15 mins
Cook: 45 mins
Serves: 8

INGREDIENTS

- 1 ½ teaspoons olive oil
- 1 pound ground turkey
- 1 onion, chopped
- 2 cups water
- 1 (28 ounce) can canned crushed tomatoes
- 1 (16 ounce) can canned kidney beans - drained, rinsed, and mashed
- 1 tablespoon garlic, minced
- 2 tablespoons chili powder
- ½ teaspoon paprika
- ½ teaspoon dried oregano
- ½ teaspoon ground cayenne pepper
- ½ teaspoon ground cumin
- ½ teaspoon salt
- ½ teaspoon ground black pepper

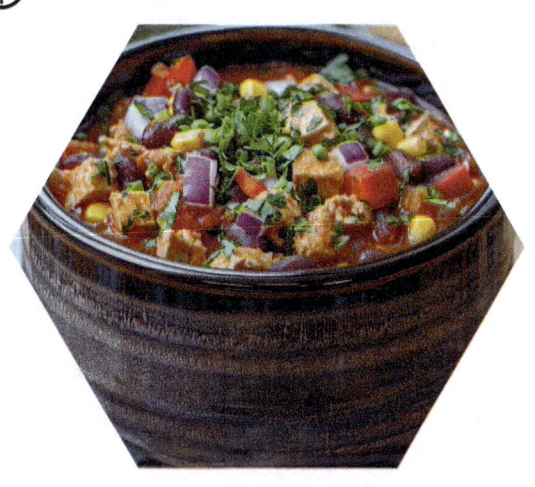

NUTRITION

- Calories: 185
- Fat: 6g
- Carbs: 19g
- Protein: 16g

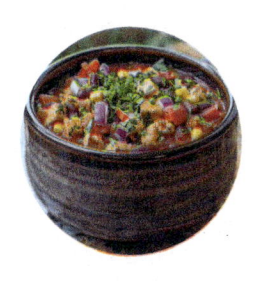

DIRECTION

1. Gather all ingredients.
2. Heat oil in a large pot over medium heat. Add turkey; cook and stir until evenly browned, 6 to 8 minutes. Stir in onion and cook until tender.
3. Add water; mix in tomatoes, kidney beans, and garlic.
4. Stir in chili powder, paprika, oregano, cayenne pepper, cumin, salt, and pepper.
5. Bring to a boil. Reduce heat to low, cover, and simmer for 30 minutes.

BARLEY, CHICKEN & MUSHROOM RISOTTO

Prep: 15 mins
Cook: 15 mins
Serves: 6

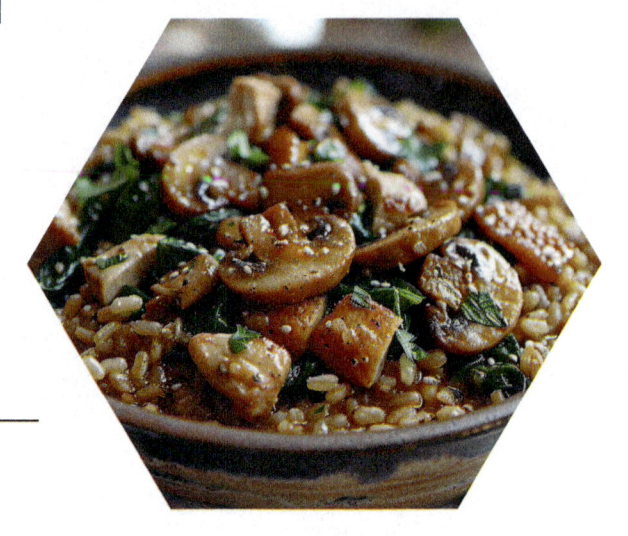

NUTRITION

- kcal: 564
- fat: 12g
- saturates: 5g
- carbs: 61g
- sugars: 3g
- fibre: 3g
- protein: 42g
- salt: 1.1g

INGREDIENTS

- 1 tbsp butter
- 1 tbsp olive oil
- 2 large shallots, finely sliced
- 1 garlic clove, chopped
- 3 skinless chicken breasts, cut into chunky pieces
- 300g pearl barley
- 250ml white wine
- 400g mixed wild and chestnut mushroom, chopped
- 1 tbsp thyme leaf
- 1l hot chicken stock
- 3 tbsp grated parmesan
- snipped chives, to serve (optional)

parmesan shavings, to serve (optional)

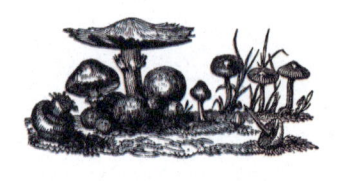

DIRECTION

1 In a large heavy saucepan, heat the butter and oil. Sauté the shallots and garlic with some seasoning for 5 mins, then stir in the chicken and cook for 2 mins.

2 Add the barley and cook for 1 min. Pour in the wine and stir until it is absorbed. Add the mushrooms and thyme, then pour over ¾ of the stock. Cook for 40 mins on a low simmer until the barley is tender, stirring occasionally and topping up with remaining stock if it looks dry. Remove from the heat and stir in the grated Parmesan. Serve immediately, with chives and Parmesan shavings scattered over, if you like.

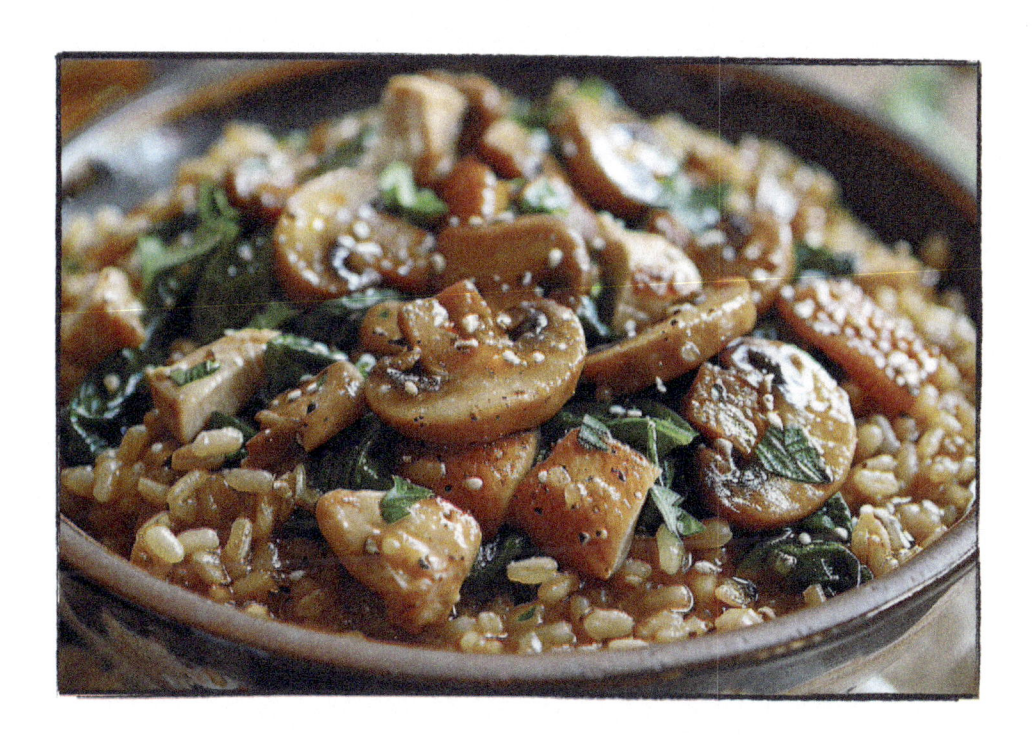

MARINATED GRILLED PORK TENDERLOIN

Prep: 10 mins
Cook: 20 mins

Serves: 4

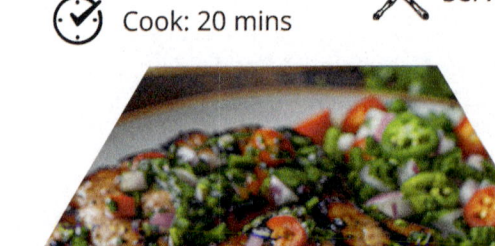

NUTRITION

- Calories: 313
- Fat: 8g
- Carbs: 28g
- Protein: 32g

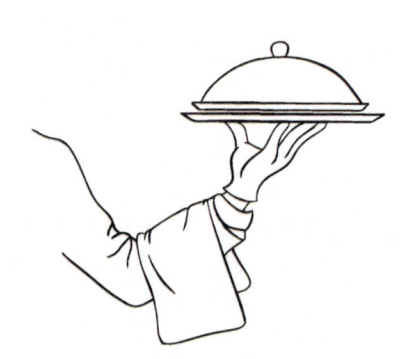

INGREDIENTS

- ¼ cup honey
- ¼ cup soy sauce
- ¼ cup oyster sauce
- 2 tablespoons brown sugar
- 4 teaspoons minced fresh ginger root
- 1 tablespoon ketchup
- 1 tablespoon minced garlic
- 1 tablespoon chopped fresh parsley
- ¼ teaspoon onion powder
- ¼ teaspoon cayenne pepper
- ¼ teaspoon ground cinnamon

DIRECTION

1. Make marinade: Whisk together honey, soy sauce, oyster sauce, brown sugar, ginger, ketchup, garlic, parsley, onion powder, cayenne pepper, and cinnamon in a medium bowl; pour into a resealable plastic bag.
2. Place pork tenderloins into the bag; coat with marinade, squeeze out excess air, and seal the bag. Marinate in the refrigerator for at least 1 hour or up to 24 hours.
3. Preheat the grill for medium heat and lightly oil the grate.
4. Remove pork tenderloins from marinade; shake off excess. Discard remaining marinade.
5. Cook pork tenderloins on the preheated grill until no longer pink in the center, 20 to 30 minutes, turning occasionally. An instant-read thermometer inserted into the centers should read at least 145 degrees F (63 degrees C).

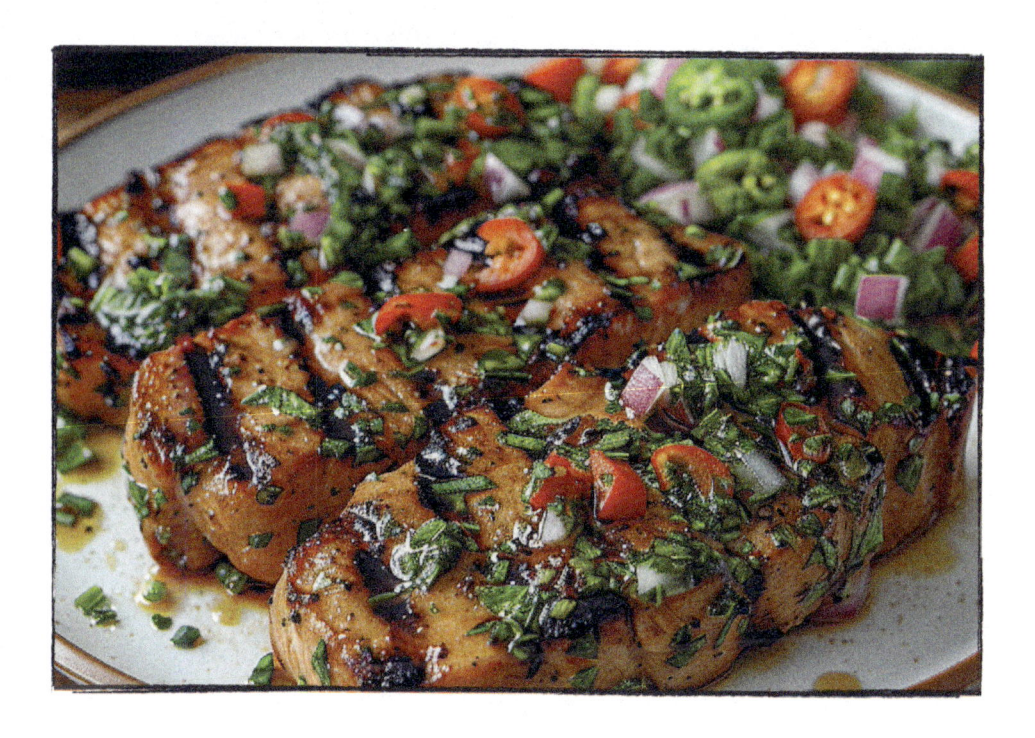

GRILLED BALSAMIC AND SOY MARINATED FLANK STEAK

Prep: 10 mins
Cook: 15 mins

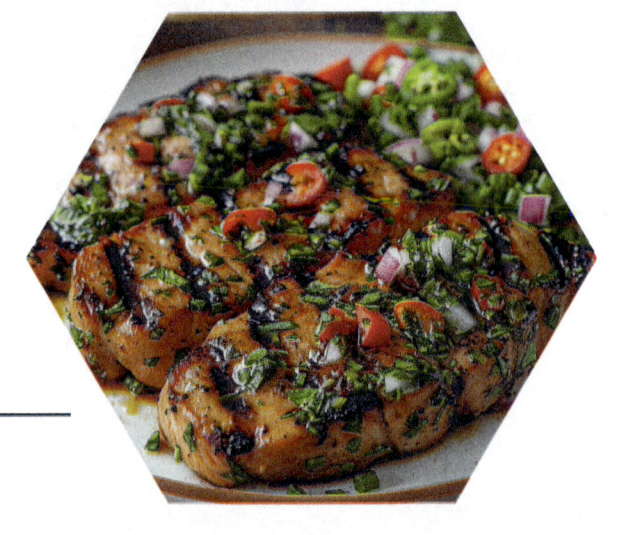

Serves: 4

NUTRITION

- Calories: 307
- Fat: 21g
- Carbs: 8g
- Protein: 22g

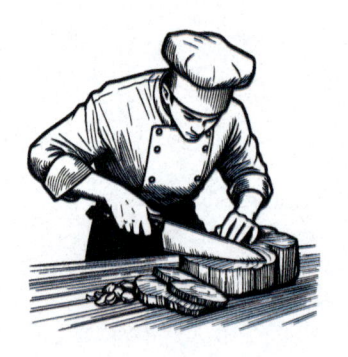

INGREDIENTS

- ½ onion, chopped
- 3 cloves garlic, chopped
- ¼ cup olive oil
- ¼ cup balsamic vinegar
- ¼ cup soy sauce
- 1 tablespoon Dijon mustard
- 1 tablespoon rosemary
- 1 teaspoon salt
- ½ teaspoon ground black pepper
- 1 ½ pounds flank steak

DIRECTION

1. Whisk onion, garlic, olive oil, balsamic vinegar, soy sauce, Dijon mustard, rosemary, salt, and pepper together in a mixing bowl.
2. Place flank steak into a large resealable plastic bag. Pour marinade into the bag and coat steak with the marinade. Squeeze excess air from the bag and seal. Marinate in the refrigerator at least 30 minutes, up to 2 days.
3. Preheat an outdoor grill for medium-high heat and lightly oil the grate.
4. Remove steak from marinade and shake to remove excess liquid. Reserve marinade.
5. Cook steak until firm, hot in the center, and just turning from pink to grey, 6 to 8 minutes per side, brushing occasionally with reserved marinade. An instant-read thermometer inserted into the center should read 150 degrees F (65 degrees C). Remove steak to a cutting board and rest meat 5 minutes before slicing thinly across the grain.

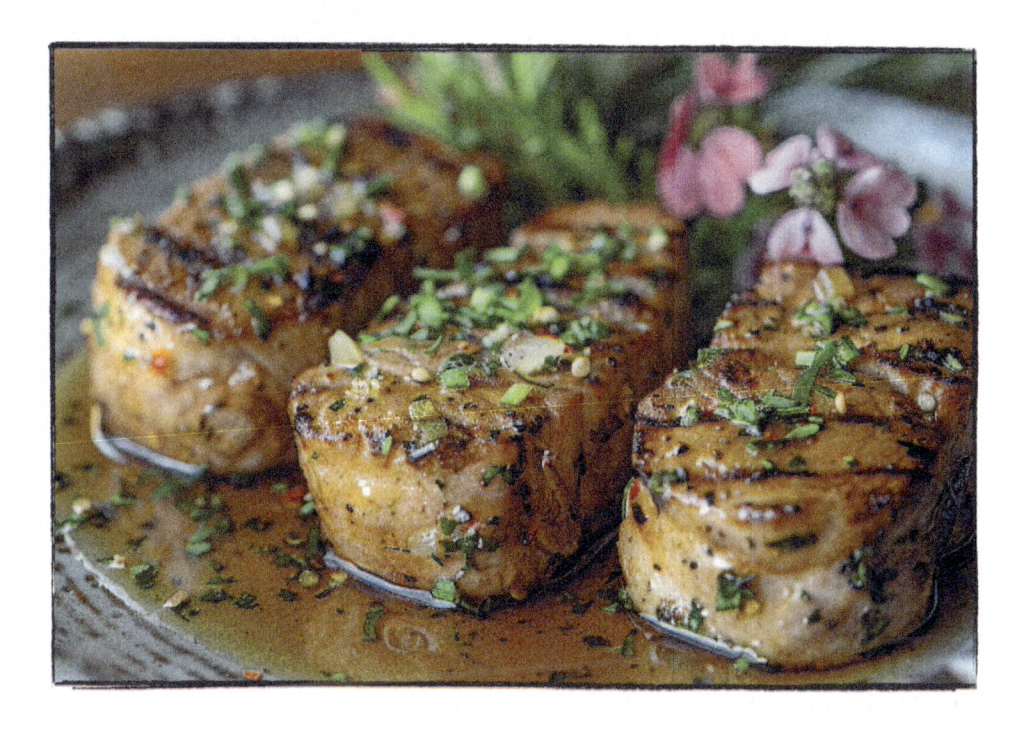

GRILLED PORTOBELLO MUSHROOMS

Prep: 10 mins
Cook: 10 mins
Serves: 3

INGREDIENTS

- 3 large portobello mushrooms
- ¼ cup canola oil
- ¼ cup balsamic vinegar, or to taste
- 3 tablespoons chopped onion
- 4 cloves garlic, minced

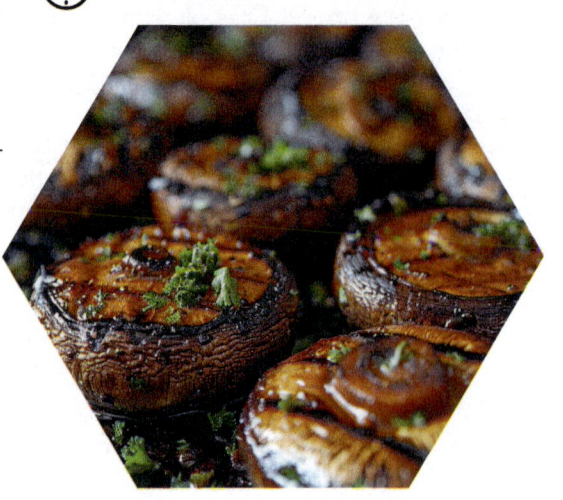

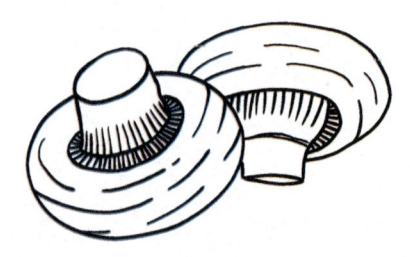

NUTRITION

- Calories: 217
- Fat: 19g
- Carbs: 11g
- Protein: 3g

DIRECTION

1. Clean mushrooms; remove stems, reserving them for another use. Place mushroom caps gill-side up in a shallow dish.
2. Combine oil, balsamic vinegar, onion, and garlic in a small bowl. Pour mixture evenly over mushroom caps; let marinate at room temperature for 1 hour.
3. Preheat the grill to medium-high heat; grease the grate.
4. Grill over the hot grill until caramelized and tender, about 5 minutes per side; serve warm.

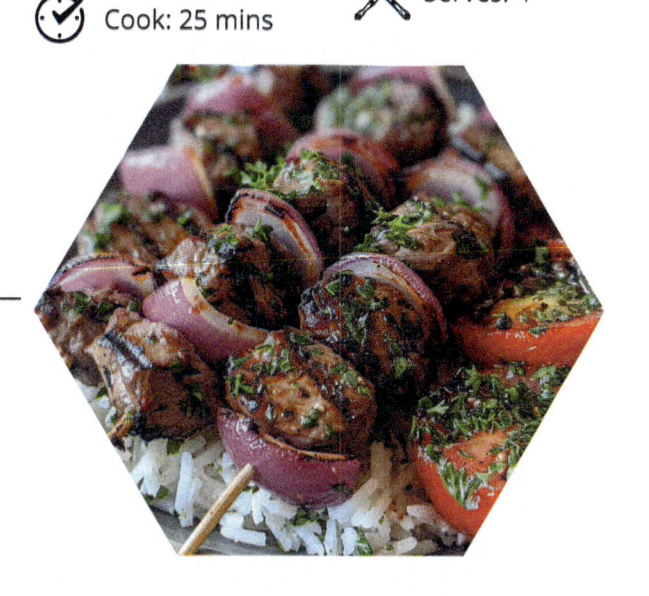

BEEF SHISH KABOBS

Prep: 20 mins
Cook: 25 mins
Serves: 4

NUTRITION

- kcal: 564
- fat: 12g
- saturates: 5g
- carbs: 61g
- sugars: 3g
- fibre: 3g
- protein: 42g
- salt: 1.1g

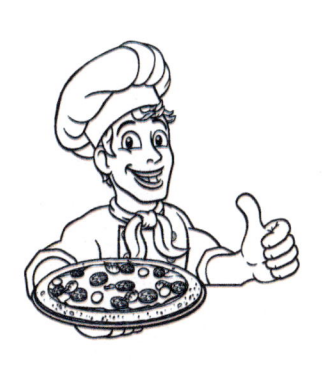

INGREDIENTS

- ½ cup soy sauce
- ⅓ cup vegetable oil
- ¼ cup lemon juice
- 1 clove garlic, minced
- 1 tablespoon prepared mustard
- 1 tablespoon Worcestershire sauce
- 1 ½ teaspoons salt, or to taste
- 1 teaspoon coarsely cracked black pepper
- 1 ½ pounds lean beef, cut into 1-inch cubes
- 16 mushroom caps
- 8 metal skewers, or as needed
- 2 green bell peppers, cut into chunks
- 1 red bell pepper, cut into chunks
- 1 large onion, cut into large squares

DIRECTION

1. Whisk together soy sauce, vegetable oil, lemon juice, garlic, mustard, Worcestershire sauce, salt, and black pepper in a bowl to make the marinade. Pour the marinade into a resealable plastic bag.
2. Add beef cubes to the bag, squeeze out excess air, and seal. Marinate in the refrigerator for 8 hours or overnight.
3. After the initial marinating time, add mushrooms to the bag, squeeze out excess air, and reseal. Marinate in the refrigerator for another 8 hours.
4. Preheat an outdoor grill for high heat and lightly oil the grate.
5. Remove beef and mushrooms from the marinade, shaking off any excess liquid. Pour the marinade into a small saucepan and bring to a boil. Reduce heat to medium-low and simmer for 10 minutes; set aside for basting.
6. Thread pieces of green bell pepper, beef, red bell pepper, mushroom, and onion onto metal skewers, repeating until all ingredients are skewered.
7. Cook the skewers on the preheated grill, turning frequently and brushing generously with the marinade prepared for basting, until nicely browned on all sides and beef is no longer pink in the center, about 15 minutes.

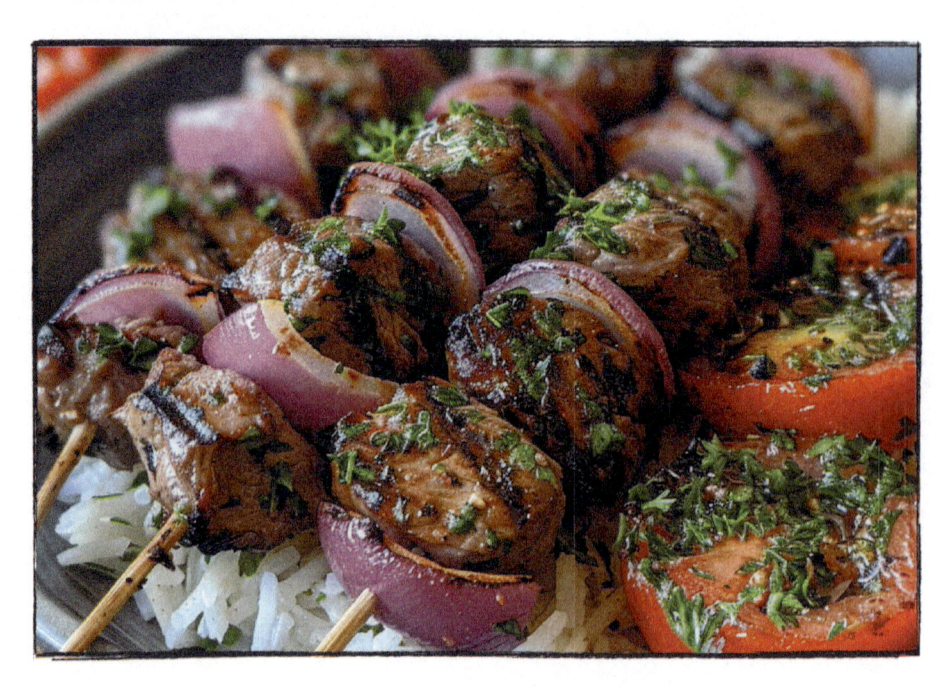

GRILLED CHICKEN WRAPS

🕐 Prep: 10 mins
✅ Cook: 10 mins

🍴 Serves: 5

INGREDIENTS

- 6 skinless, boneless chicken breast halves
- 4 links pork sausage
- 2 jalapeno peppers, seeded and minced
- ¾ cup chopped onion
- 3 cloves garlic, chopped
- 1 teaspoon Cajun seasoning
- 12 slices bacon

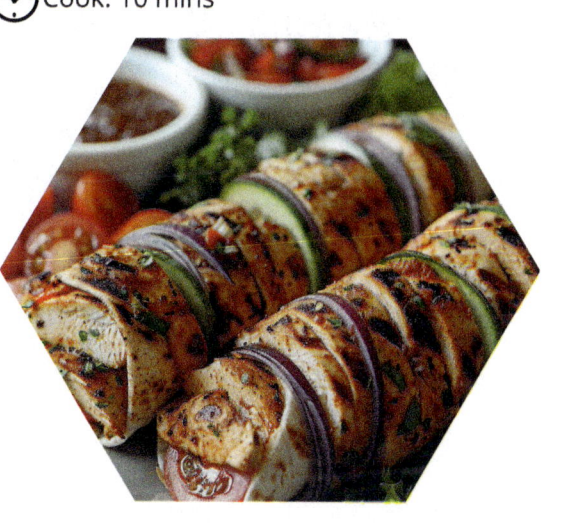

NUTRITION

- Calories: 531
- Fat: 36g
- Carbs: 4g
- Protein: 44g

DIRECTION

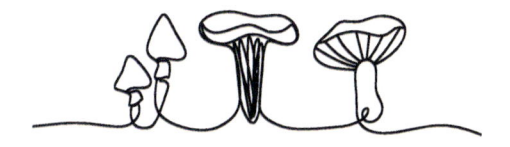

1. Slit open each chicken breast. Cut each sausage link in half lengthways, then cut to the length of the chicken breast. Place a halved sausage link inside each chicken breast, then add jalapeno peppers to taste, onion and garlic and seal the chicken with toothpicks.
2. Season the outside of each chicken breast with Cajun spices/seasoning. Wrap each breast with 2 slices of bacon and secure with toothpicks. Place on a barbecue grill over medium coals and grill until done, about 30 minutes each side. Enjoy!

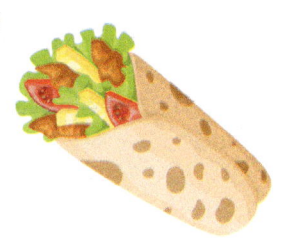

ASPARAGUS WITH SLICED ALMONDS AND PARMESAN CHEESE

Prep: 10 mins
Cook: 10 mins

Serves: 5

INGREDIENTS

- 2 tablespoons butter
- 1 pound asparagus, bottoms trimmed
- ⅓ cup sliced almonds
- ⅓ cup Parmesan cheese

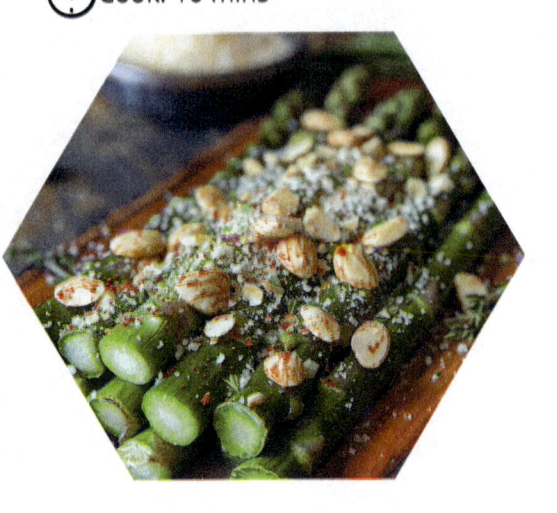

NUTRITION

- Calories: 178
- Fat: 14g
- Carbs: 7g
- Protein: 8g

DIRECTION

Melt butter in a large skillet over medium-high heat. Add the asparagus, and cook, stirring, about 3 minutes. Stir in almonds and parmesan, and cook until the cheese is slightly browned, about 3 to 5 minutes.

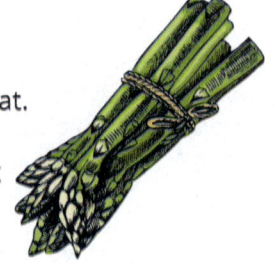

VEGETARIAN SCRAMBLED EGGS

Prep: 10 mins
Cook: 15 mins
Serves: 6

INGREDIENTS

- ¼ cup olive oil
- ¼ cup sliced fresh mushrooms
- ¼ cup chopped onions
- ¼ cup chopped green bell peppers
- 6 eggs
- ¼ cup milk
- ¼ cup chopped fresh tomato
- ¼ cup shredded Cheddar cheese

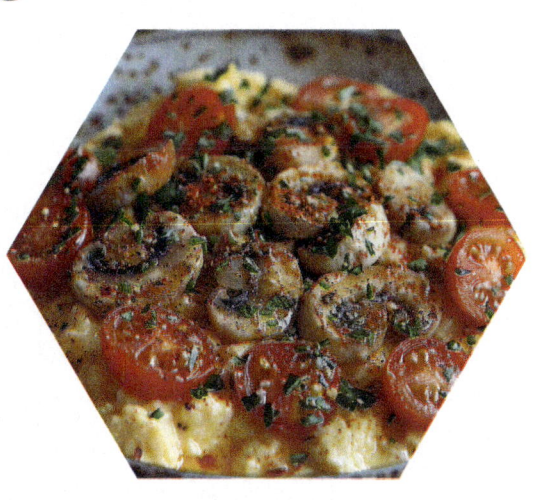

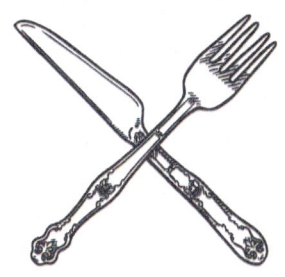

NUTRITION

- Calories: 313
- Fat: 1g
- Carbs: 79g
- Protein: 3g

DIRECTION

1. Heat olive oil in a skillet or frying pan over medium-high heat. Add mushrooms, onions and peppers; saute until onions are transparent.
2. In a mixing bowl, beat together eggs and milk. Add egg mixture to vegetables; stir in tomatoes. Cook until eggs are set. When eggs are almost done, mix in cheese. Serve immediately.

CHICKEN PHO

🕐 Prep: 10 mins
✓ Cook: 30 hr

🍴 Serves: 2

NUTRITION

- Calories: 521
- Fat: 14g
- Carbs: 54g
- Protein: 50g

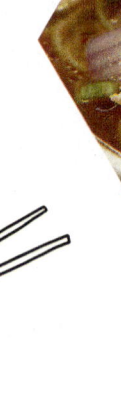

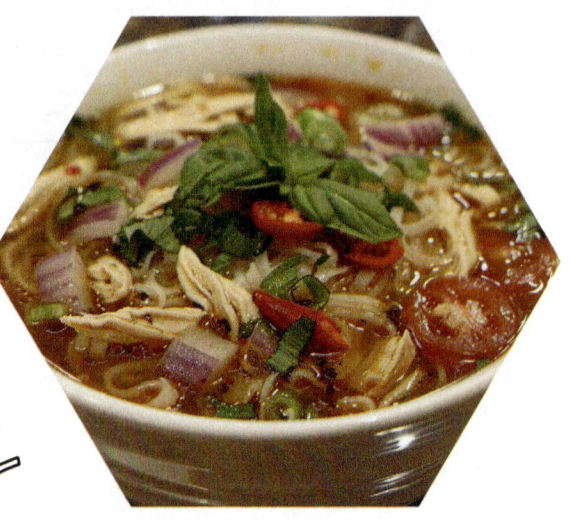

INGREDIENTS

- 4 ounces dry Chinese egg noodles
- 6 cups chicken stock
- 2 tablespoons fish sauce
- 4 cloves garlic, minced
- 2 teaspoons minced fresh ginger root
- 1 tablespoon minced lemon grass
- 5 green onions, chopped
- 2 cups cubed cooked chicken
- 1 cup bean sprouts
- 1 cup chopped bok choy

DIRECTION

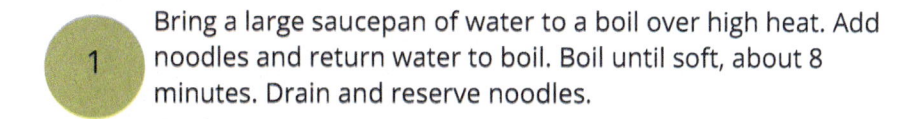

1 Bring a large saucepan of water to a boil over high heat. Add noodles and return water to boil. Boil until soft, about 8 minutes. Drain and reserve noodles.

2 Bring chicken stock, fish sauce, garlic, ginger, lemon grass, and green onions to a boil in a large pot. Reduce to a simmer; cook for 10 minutes. Stir in the chicken, bean sprouts, and bok choy. Cook pho until heated through, about 5 minutes.

3 Divide the cooked noodles between 2 large bowls. Pour pho over noodles; serve immediately.

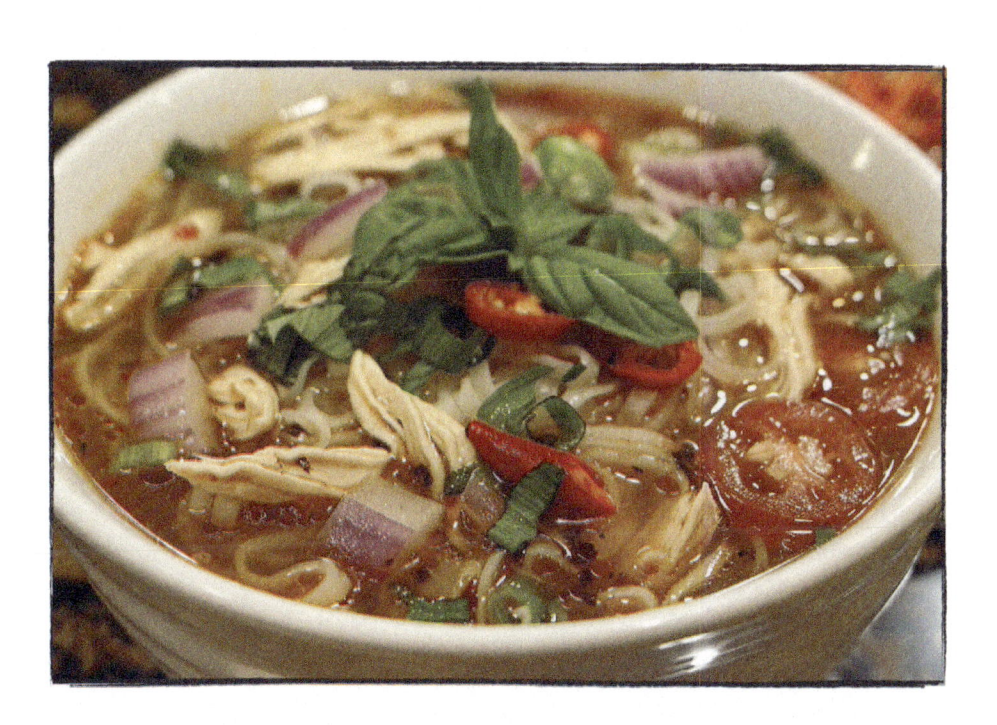

SIMPLE PEANUT BUTTER BANANA BREAD

Prep: 20 mins
Cook: 10 hr
Serves: 10

INGREDIENTS

- ¾ cup peanut butter
- ⅓ cup shortening
- ⅔ cup white sugar
- 1 cup mashed very ripe banana
- 2 eggs
- 1 ¾ cups all-purpose flour
- 2 teaspoons baking powder
- ½ teaspoon salt
- ¼ teaspoon baking soda
- ¼ cup buttermilk

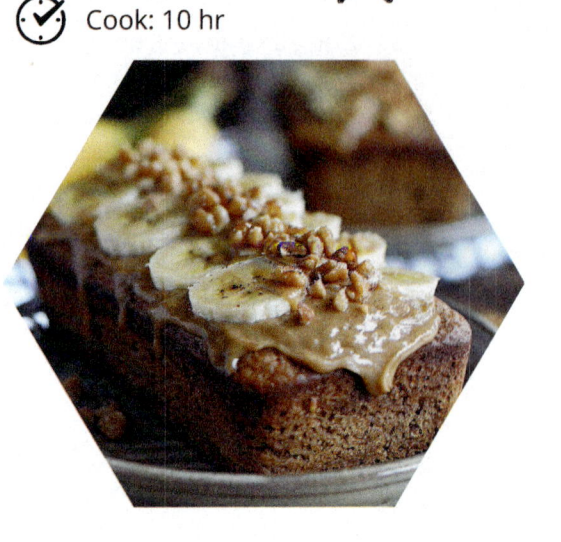

NUTRITION

- Calories: 336
- Fat: 18g
- Carbs: 38g
- Protein: 9g

DIRECTION

1. Preheat oven to 350 degrees F (175 degrees C). Grease a 4x8-inch loaf pan.
2. Beat peanut butter and shortening in a bowl. Gradually add sugar, beating until light and fluffy. Beat one egg into peanut butter mixture until completely blended before beating in the second egg. Stir in mashed banana.
3. Combine flour, baking powder, salt, and baking soda in a bowl. Stir flour mixture into banana mixture alternately with buttermilk, mixing until batter is just blended. Pour batter into prepared loaf pan.
4. Bake in the preheated oven until a toothpick inserted into the center comes out clean, about 1 hour.

WHOLE GRAIN PANCAKES TOPPED WITH FRUIT

Prep: 15 mins
Cook: 20 mins
Serves: 4

INGREDIENTS

- ¾ cup all-purpose flour
- ¾ cup whole wheat flour
- 1 ½ teaspoons baking powder
- ½ teaspoon salt
- 1 cup 2% milk
- 2 large eggs, slightly beaten
- 2 tablespoons Country Crock® Spread, plus additional for cooking and serving
- 2 cups fresh fruit (such as blueberries, bananas, and strawberries)
- Maple syrup

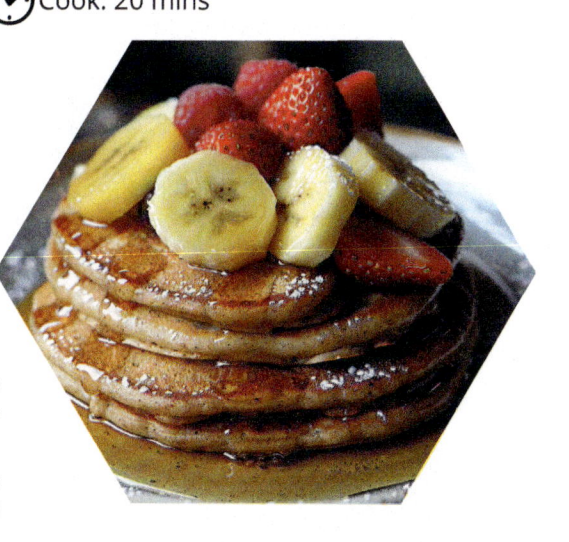

NUTRITION

- Calories: 252
- Fat: 5g
- Carbs: 43g
- Protein: 11g

DIRECTION

1. Combine flours, baking powder, and salt in a large bowl.
2. In a medium bowl, beat together milk, eggs, and 2 tablespoons melted Country Crock® Spread with a wire whisk.
3. Slowly whisk the milk mixture into the flour mixture until just combined; set aside.
4. Melt 1 tablespoon of Country Crock® Spread in a skillet.
5. Drop batter by 1/4-cupfuls into the skillet and cook pancakes, turning once, until done.
6. Repeat with remaining batter, adding additional Spread to the skillet as needed.
7. Serve pancakes topped with additional Spread, fresh fruit, and maple syrup.

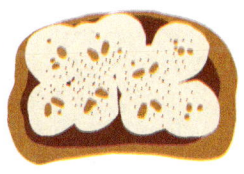

COTTAGE CHEESE TOAST

🕙 Prep: 10 mins
✓ Cook: 5 mins

🍴 Serves: 4

NUTRITION

- Calories: 174
- Fat: 1g
- Carbs: 32g
- Protein: 9g

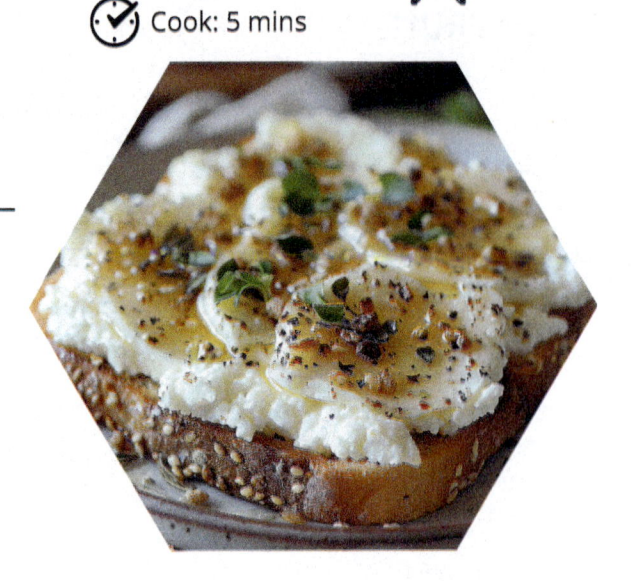

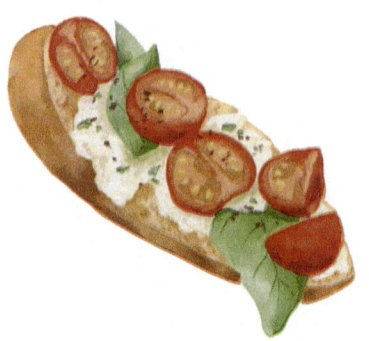

INGREDIENTS

- 1 cup low-fat cottage cheese
- 4 slices crusty Italian bread
- 1/2 cup chopped strawberries
- 1/2 cup blackberries, halved
- 4 tablespoons honey, or as needed

DIRECTION

1. Place cottage cheese into the bowl of a food processor or blender. Blend until smooth, about 1 minute, scraping down the sides after 30 seconds.
2. Toast bread slices. Top each slice with 1/4 cup cottage cheese, then top with 1/4 cup mixed berries. Drizzle each slice with 1 tablespoon honey, or more to taste.

BROWN RICE PUDDING

Prep: 10 mins
Cook: 2hr
Serves: 4

NUTRITION

- Calories: 517
- Fat: 40g
- Carbs: 38g
- Protein: 5g

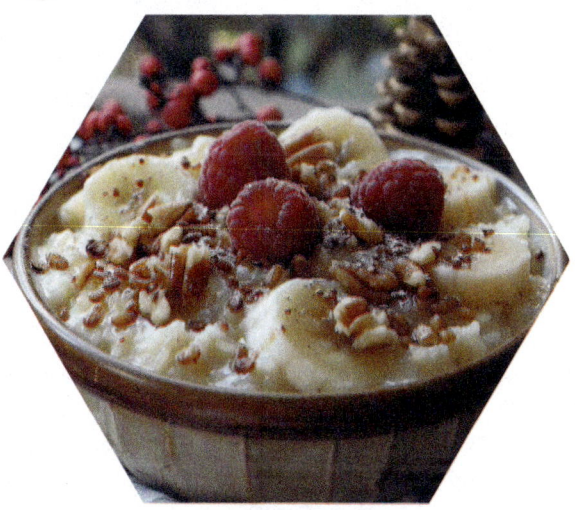

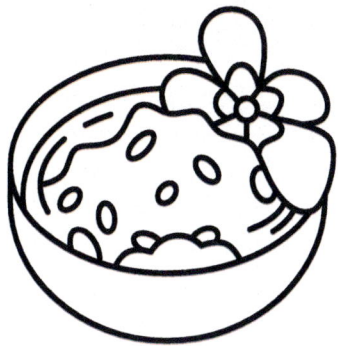

INGREDIENTS

- 1 ½ cups heavy cream
- 1 ¼ cups water
- ½ cup short-grain brown rice
- ¼ teaspoon salt
- ½ cup raisins (Optional)
- 3 egg yolks
- ¼ cup white sugar
- ½ teaspoon ground cinnamon
- 1 tablespoon butter, softened
- 2 teaspoons vanilla extract

DIRECTION

1. Bring the heavy cream, water, brown rice, and salt to a boil in a pot; reduce heat to low, cover, and simmer until the liquid is completely absorbed, about 80 minutes. Fold the raisins into the mixture and continue cooking until the raisins plump, about 10 minutes more.
2. Whisk the egg yolks, sugar, and cinnamon together in a bowl; slowly pour into the pot with the rice while stirring. Cook and stir until the mixture thickens, about 6 minutes. Remove from heat and stir in the butter and vanilla extract.

COFFEE JELLY

🕐 Prep: 5 mins
✓ Cook: 5 mins

🍴 Serves: 4

NUTRITION

- Calories: 43
- Carbs: 9g
- Protein: 2g

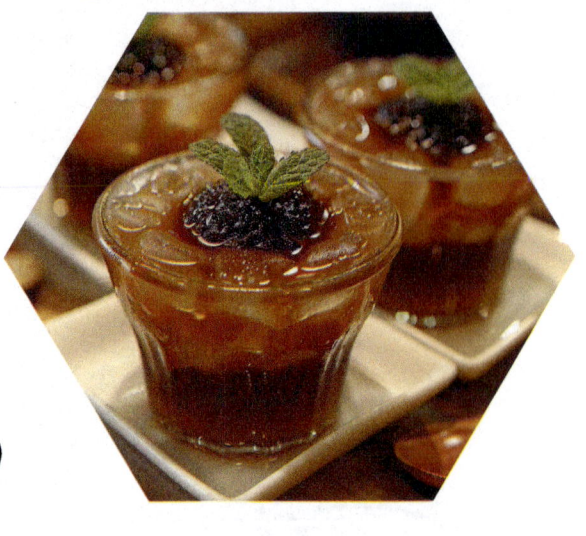

INGREDIENTS

- 2 tablespoons hot water
- 1 (.25 ounce) package unflavored gelatin
- 2 cups fresh brewed coffee
- 3 tablespoons white sugar

DIRECTION

1. Gather all ingredients.
2. Dissolve gelatin in hot water, then mix in coffee and sugar in a saucepan, bringing it to a boil.
3. Pour the mixture into a baking dish and chill until solidified in the refrigerator for 6 to 7 hours.
4. Cut the set coffee jelly into cubes.
5. Serve and enjoy!

LEMON GINGER WATER

Prep: 10 mins
Cook: 10 mins
Serves: 16

NUTRITION

- Calories: 8
- Carbs: 2g

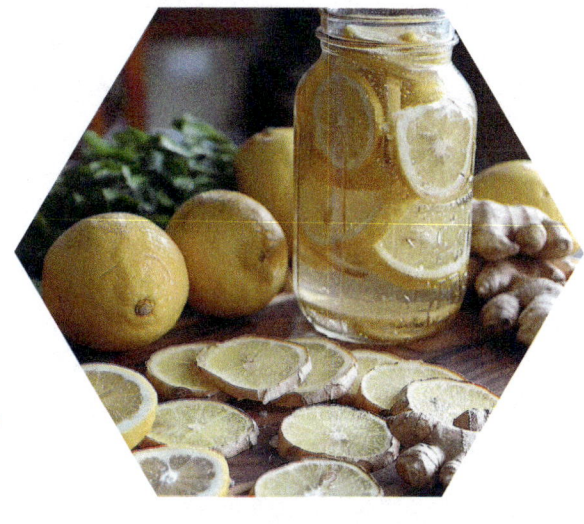

INGREDIENTS

- ½ cup lemon juice
- 15 ½ cups filtered water, divided
- 1 (2 inch) piece fresh ginger, peeled
- 4 teaspoons honey
- 4 quart-size mason jars (optional)

DIRECTION

1. Gather the ingredients.
2. Combine lemon juice, 1/2 cup water, ginger, and honey in a blender; blend for 20 to 30 seconds.
3. Strain the mixture evenly into 4 quart-sized mason jars or a 1-gallon pitcher.
4. Top off with remaining water and stir. Place lids on the jars or cover pitcher and store in the refrigerator.

CHIA SEED PUDDING

🕐 Prep: 15 mins
✓ Cook: No cook

🍴 Serves: 4

NUTRITION

- Calories: 243
- Fat: 8g
- Carbs: 38g
- Protein: 7g

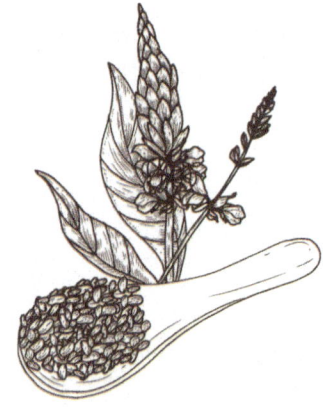

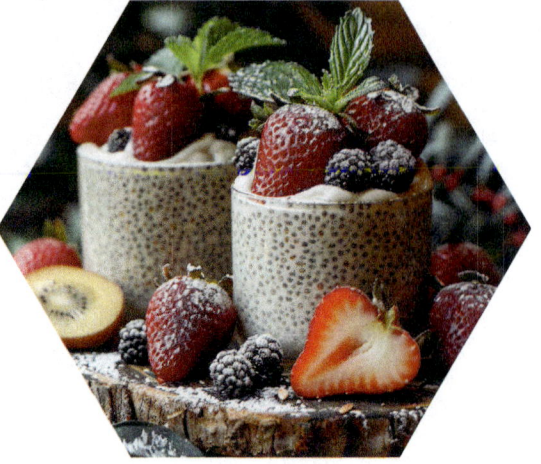

INGREDIENTS

- 1 cup unsweetened vanilla-flavored almond milk
- 1 cup vanilla fat-free yogurt
- 2 tablespoons pure maple syrup
- 1 teaspoon pure vanilla extract
- ⅛ teaspoon salt
- ¼ cup chia seeds
- 1 pint strawberries, hulled and chopped
- 4 teaspoons pure maple syrup
- ¼ cup toasted almonds

DIRECTION

1. Whisk almond milk, yogurt, 2 tablespoons maple syrup, vanilla, and salt together in a bowl until just blended; add chia seeds, whisk to incorporate, and let the chia seeds soak for 30 minutes.
2. Stir the chia seed mixture to redistribute seeds that have settled throughout the mixture. Cover the bowl with plastic wrap and refrigerate 8 hours to overnight.
3. Drizzle 4 teaspoons maple syrup over strawberries in a bowl; stir to coat. Add almonds to strawberries; stir.
4. Spoon chia seed mixture into 4 bowls; top each with a portion of the strawberry mixture.

GREEK YOGURT BOWLS WITH GRANOLA

Prep: 20 mins
Cook: 55 mins
Serves: 20

INGREDIENTS

- Walnut-Honey Mix:
- 1 cup chopped walnuts
- 1 cup light honey
- Granola:
- 2 cups rolled oats
- ¾ cup raw buckwheat groats
- ½ cup buckwheat flakes
- ½ cup chopped raw almonds
- ½ cup chopped raw hazelnuts
- ½ cup sunflower seeds
- 1 teaspoon ground cinnamon
- ½ teaspoon ground nutmeg
- ¼ teaspoon ground allspice
- ⅛ teaspoon ground ginger
- ½ cup light olive oil
- ½ cup packed coconut sugar
- ¼ cup brown rice syrup, or more to taste
- 2 teaspoons vanilla extract
- 1 cup shredded unsweetened coconut
- ½ cup coarsely ground flax seeds
- ½ cup raisins
- ¼ cup golden raisins
- Yogurt Bowls:
- 10 cups plain nonfat Greek yogurt
- 5 cups fresh raspberries

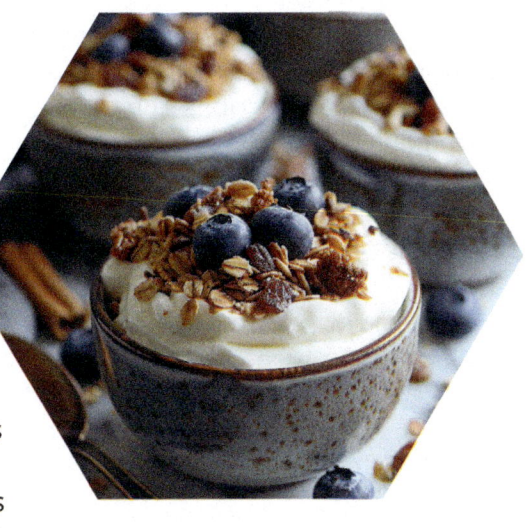

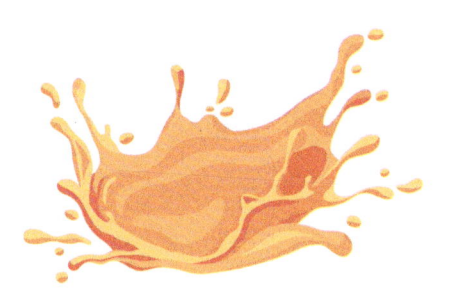

NUTRITION

- Calories: 435
- Fat: 20g
- Carbs: 53g
- Protein: 16g

DIRECTION

1. Preheat the oven to 300°F (150°C) and line 2 rimmed baking sheets with parchment paper.
2. Combine walnuts and honey in a jar, cover, and set aside.
3. In a bowl, mix oats, groats, buckwheat flakes, almonds, hazelnuts, sunflower seeds, cinnamon, nutmeg, allspice, and ginger until well combined.
4. In a small saucepan over low heat, stir together olive oil, coconut sugar, and brown rice syrup until combined and heated through (about 5 minutes). Remove from heat, stir in vanilla extract, then pour over the dry mixture and mix until evenly combined.
5. Spread the mixture evenly over the prepared baking sheets.
6. Bake in the preheated oven for 25 minutes. Stir, rotate the baking sheets, and bake for another 15 minutes. Stir again, rotate once more, and bake until golden brown for about 15 more minutes.
7. Sprinkle coconut, flax seeds, and raisins over the granola and toss to mix.
8. Turn off the oven, but leave trays inside and prop the oven door open with a wooden spoon for 10 minutes.
9. Remove from the oven and allow to cool before serving.
10. Place 1/2 cup yogurt in a deep single-serve bowl. Top with a scant 1/3 cup granola, 1/4 cup raspberries, and 1/8 cup walnut-honey mix. Repeat to assemble remaining bowls.

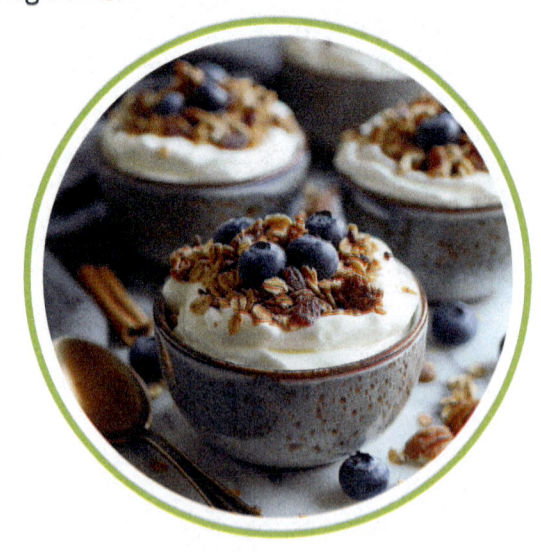

VEGAN OVERNIGHT OATS WITH CHIA SEEDS AND FRUIT

Prep: 5 mins
Cook: 5 mins
Serves: 2

NUTRITION

- Calories: 492
- Fat: 12g
- Carbs: 88g
- Protein: 13g

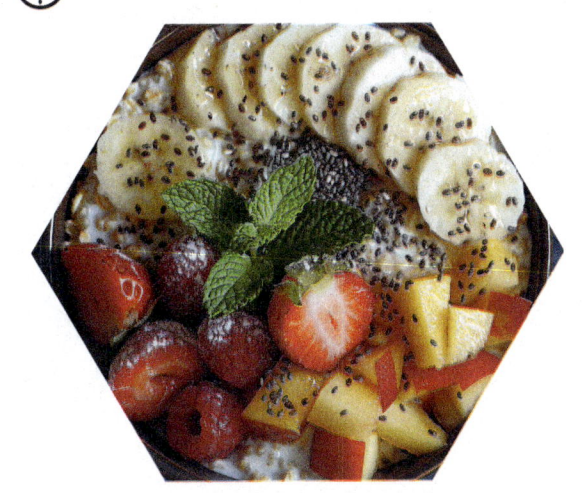

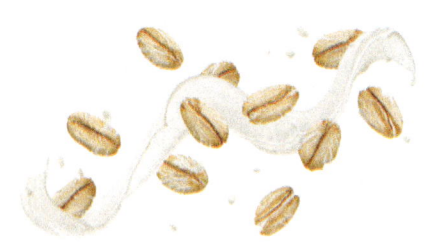

INGREDIENTS

- 1 cup unsweetened vanilla-flavored almond milk
- 1 cup vanilla fat-free yogurt
- 2 tablespoons pure maple syrup
- 1 teaspoon pure vanilla extract
- ⅛ teaspoon salt
- ¼ cup chia seeds
- 1 pint strawberries, hulled and chopped
- 4 teaspoons pure maple syrup
- ¼ cup toasted almonds

DIRECTION

1. Whisk almond milk, yogurt, 2 tablespoons maple syrup, vanilla, and salt together in a bowl until just blended; add chia seeds, whisk to incorporate, and let the chia seeds soak for 30 minutes.
2. Stir the chia seed mixture to redistribute seeds that have settled throughout the mixture. Cover the bowl with plastic wrap and refrigerate 8 hours to overnight.
3. Drizzle 4 teaspoons maple syrup over strawberries in a bowl; stir to coat. Add almonds to strawberries; stir.
4. Spoon chia seed mixture into 4 bowls; top each with a portion of the strawberry mixture.

CARROT AND ORANGE JUICE

Prep: 10 mins
Cook: 10 mins
Serves: 4

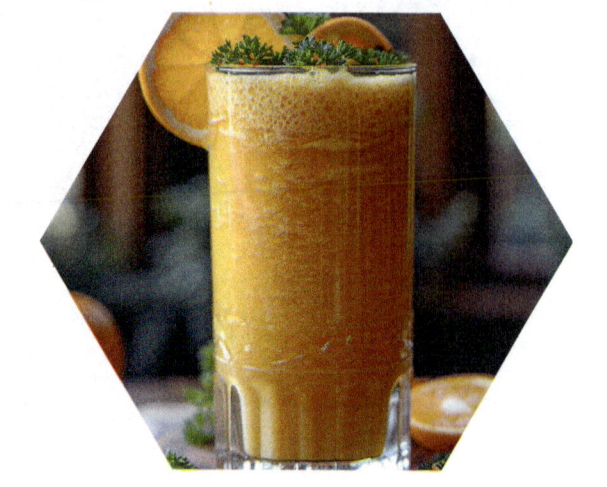

NUTRITION

- Calories: 183
- Fat: 1g
- Carbs: 44g
- Protein: 4g

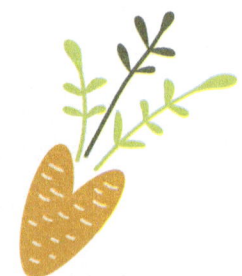

INGREDIENTS

- 2 pounds organic carrots, trimmed and scrubbed
- 8 organic oranges, peeled

DIRECTION

1. Press carrots and oranges through a juicer and into a large glass.

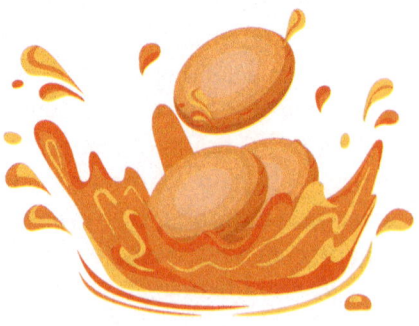

BANANA SPLIT CHIA SEED PUDDING

Prep: 10 mins
Cook: 0 mins
Serves: 4

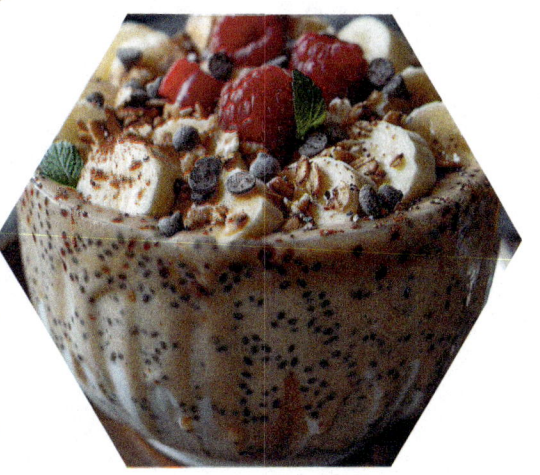

INGREDIENTS

- 1 cup Almond Breeze Unsweetened Vanilla Almondmilk
- 1/2 cup plain Greek yogurt
- 1 1/2 tablespoons pure maple syrup
- 1/2 teaspoon vanilla extract
- 1/4 cup chia seeds
- 1 banana, thinly sliced
- 1/2 cup chopped strawberries
- 1/2 cup blueberries
- 1/4 cup unsweetened coconut flakes, toasted
- 2 tablespoons cacao nibs

NUTRITION

- Calories: 307
- Fat: 21g
- Carbs: 8g
- Protein: 22g

DIRECTION

1. Stir together Almond Breeze Unsweetened Vanilla Almondmilk, Greek yogurt, maple syrup and vanilla in a container with a lid. Whisk in chia seeds. Cover and refrigerate for at least 4 hours, best overnight.
2. When you're ready to eat the chia pudding, prepare the toppings. Preheat a sauté pan to medium heat. Add coconut flakes and stir constantly until they turn a golden color, 1 to 3 minutes. Remove coconut flakes from the pan and allow to cool.
3. Stir chia seed pudding to make sure there aren't any big clumps, then spoon into 4 serving dishes. Top evenly with banana slices, strawberries, blueberries, coconut flakes and cacao nibs.

BAKED CINNAMON APPLES

Prep: 10 mins
Cook: 45 mins

Serves: 4

NUTRITION

- Calories: 173
- Fat: 2g
- Carbs: 41g
- Protein: 1g

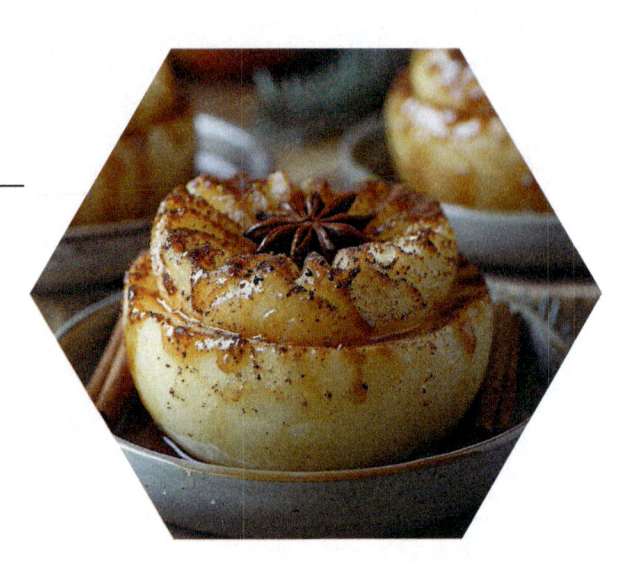

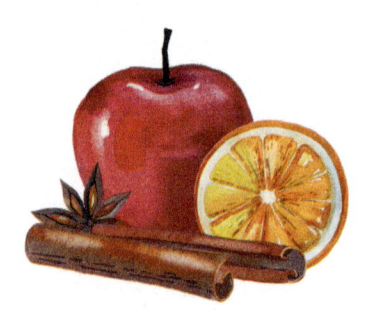

INGREDIENTS

- 3 Golden Delicious apples - peeled, cored, and thinly sliced
- ⅔ cup water
- 2 teaspoons cold butter, cut into small pieces
- 1 ½ teaspoons all-purpose flour
- 1 teaspoon cornstarch
- ½ cup brown sugar
- ¼ teaspoon ground cinnamon
- 1 pinch salt

DIRECTION

1 Preheat the oven to 350 degrees F (175 degrees C).

2 Layer apple slices on the bottom of an 8-inch glass baking dish.

3 Bring chicken stock, fish sauce, garlic, ginger, lemon grass, and green onions to a boil in a large pot. Reduce to a simmer; cook for 10 minutes. Stir in the chicken, bean sprouts, and bok choy. Cook pho until heated through, about 5 minutes.

4 Divide the cooked noodles between 2 large bowls. Pour pho over noodles; serve immediately.

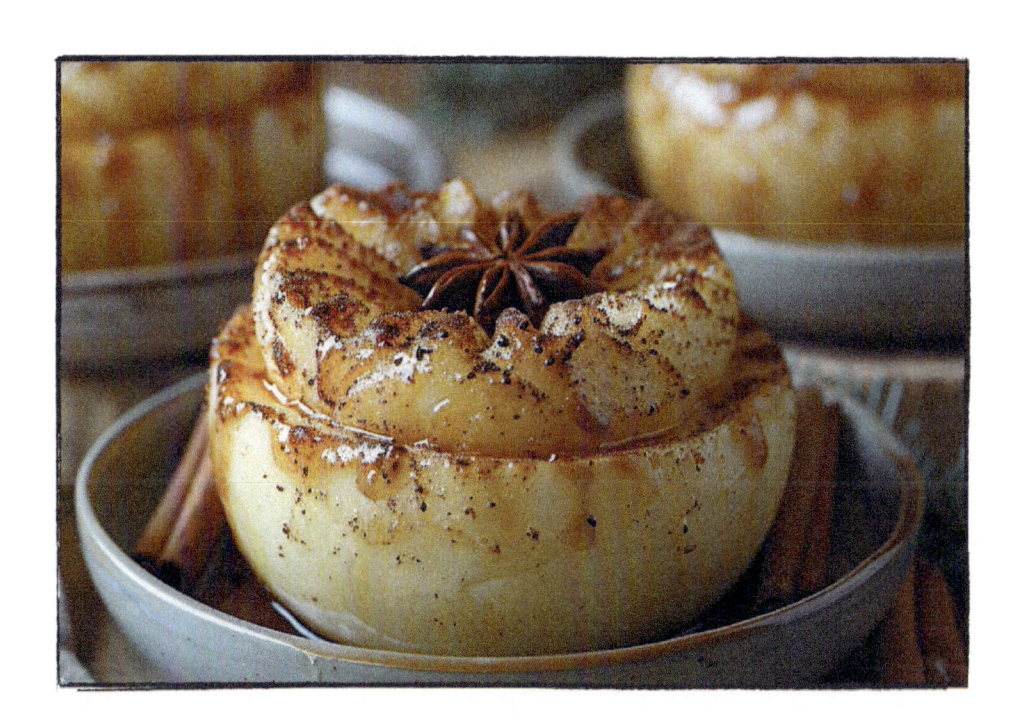

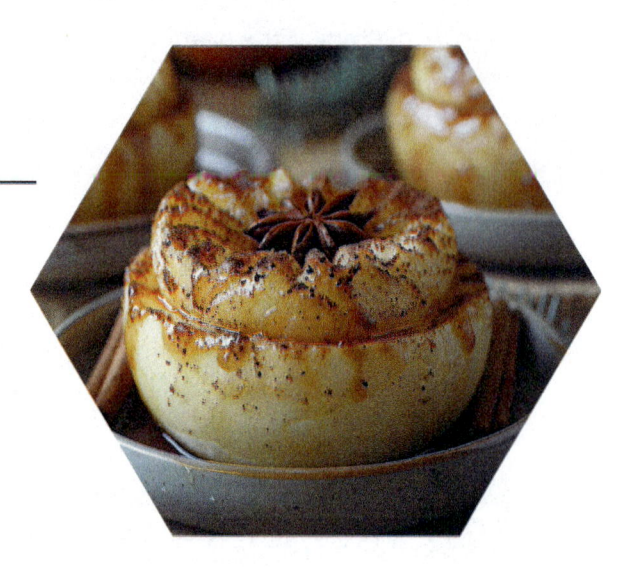

RATATOUILLE

Prep: 15 mins
Cook: 45 mins

Serves: 4

NUTRITION

- kcal: 261
- fat: 15g
- saturates: 2g
- carbs: 19g
- sugars: 17g
- fibre: 11g
- protein: 6g
- salt: 0.03g

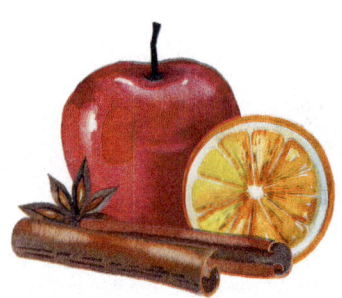

INGREDIENTS

- 2 large aubergines
- 4 small courgettes
- 2 red or yellow peppers
- 4 large ripe tomatoes
- 5 tbsp olive oil
- supermarket pack or small bunch basil
- 1 medium onion, peeled and thinly sliced
- 3 garlic cloves, peeled and crushed
- 1 tbsp red wine vinegar

1 tsp sugar (any kind)

DIRECTION

1 Preheat the oven to 350 degrees F (175 degrees C). Coat the bottom and sides of a 1 1/2-quart casserole dish with 1 tablespoon olive oil.

2 Heat remaining 1 tablespoon olive oil in a medium skillet over medium heat. Cook and stir garlic until fragrant and golden brown. Add eggplant and parsley; cook and stir until eggplant is tender and soft, about 10 minutes. Season with salt to taste.

3 Spread eggplant mixture evenly across the bottom of the prepared casserole dish; sprinkle with a few tablespoons of Parmesan cheese. Spread zucchini in an even layer over top. Lightly salt and sprinkle with a little more cheese. Continue layering in this fashion, with tomatoes, mushrooms, onion, and bell pepper, covering each layer with a sprinkling of salt and cheese.

4 Bake in preheated oven until vegetables are tender, about 45 minutes.

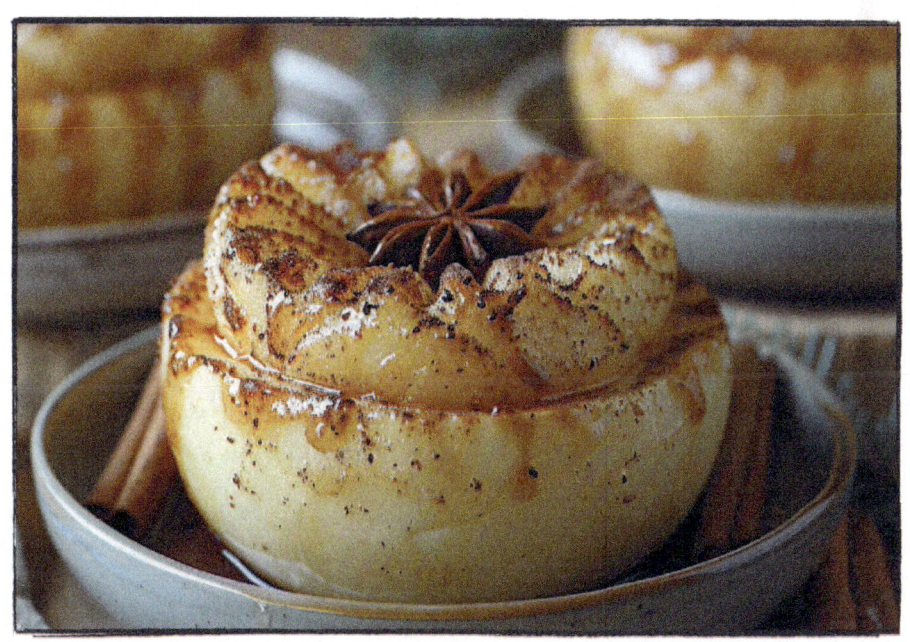

CREAMY GARLIC, LEMON & SPINACH SALMON

Prep: 10 mins
Cook: 0 mins
Serves: 4

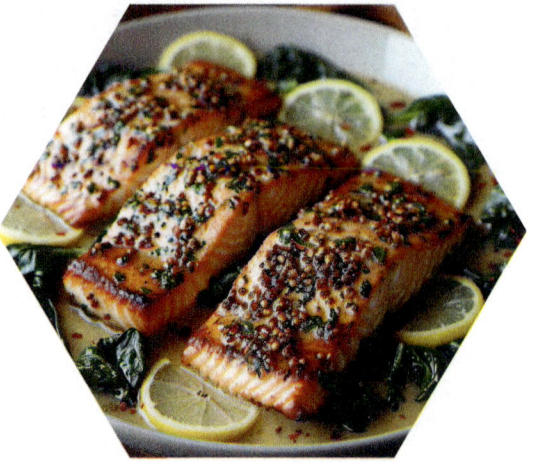

INGREDIENTS

- 2 sweet potatoes
- 1 tbsp olive oil or rapeseed oil
- 2 salmon fillets, skin removed
- 2 garlic cloves, thinly sliced
- 170g baby spinach
- 1 lemon, zested and ½ juiced, ½ thinly sliced
- 75g mascarpone

5 tbsp milk

NUTRITION

- kcal: 721
- fat: 44g
- saturates: 16g
- carbs: 34g
- sugars: 19g
- fibre: 7g
- protein: 43g
- salt: 0.5g

DIRECTION

1. Preheat the oven to 200°C (180°C fan/gas 6). Microwave the pierced sweet potatoes for 5 minutes or bake for 35-40 minutes until soft.
2. Lightly brown the salmon in a pan with some oil. Sauté garlic, then add spinach, lemon zest, and juice to the same pan. Mix in mascarpone and some milk until the spinach wilts.
3. Place the spinach mixture in an ovenproof dish, top with lemon slices and salmon fillets. Bake for 5-8 minutes until the salmon is cooked through.
4. Scoop out and mash the sweet potato flesh with the remaining milk and season. Serve the mashed sweet potatoes alongside the creamy spinach and salmon.

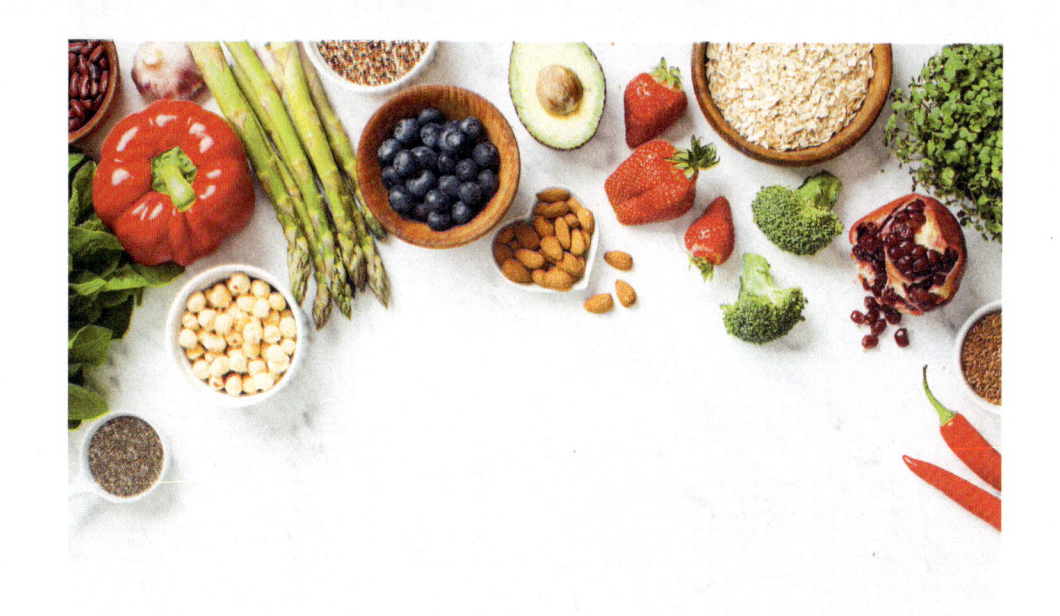

GOOD HEALTH

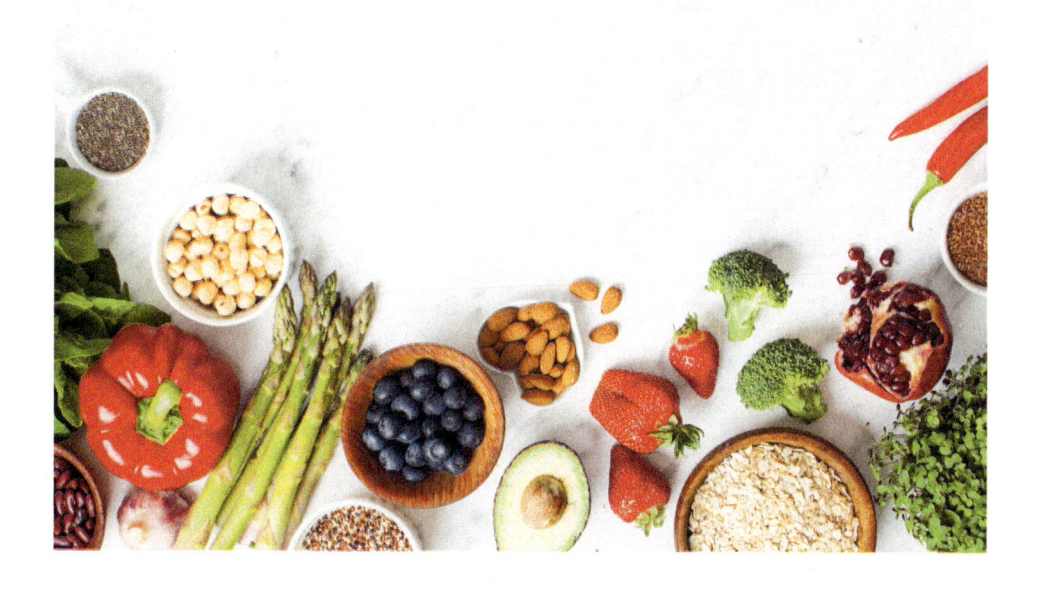

Printed in Great Britain
by Amazon